THE

HAPPY HORMONE

GUIDE

A PLANT-BASED PROGRAM
TO BALANCE HORMONES, INCREASE
ENERGY, & REDUCE PMS SYMPTOMS

SHANNON LEPARSKI

Copyright ©2019 by Shannon Leparski
Published by Blue Star Press
PO Box 8835, Bend, OR 97708
contact@bluestarpress.com | www.bluestarpress.com

Photography by:
Shannon Leparski: Cover and pages 4, 47, 59, 68, 77, 85, 131, 135, 137, 139, 140, 143-144, 147, 154, 157-160, 163-164, 167-168, 181-184, 187, 189-191, 206-213
and
Sara Hilton: pages 9, 16-17, 27, 41, 44, 65, 75, 92-93, 107

Cover Design: Amanda Hudson
Interior Design: Amy Sly

ISBN 9781944515836

Printed in Colombia

10 9 8 7 6 5 4

DISCLAIMER:
This book is for informational and educational purposes. Please consult your healthcare provider before beginning any healthcare program.

*To the ladies looking for alternative methods
to balance your hormones.*

Also, don't worry—it's just a phase.

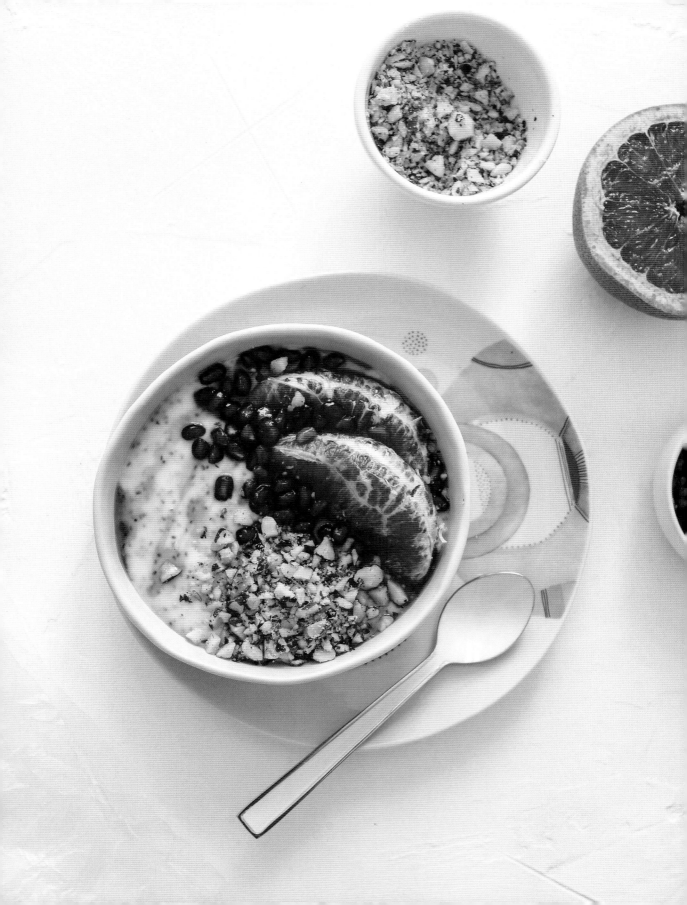

CONTENTS

INTRODUCTION

*My Journey to
Happy Hormones*

SOMETIMES LIVING IN A WOMAN'S BODY CAN feel like riding a roller coaster in the dark. It's a shaky, loopy journey and you can't always tell where you are heading next. I vividly remember my stomach doing somersaults after coming home from school in the seventh grade to find I had started my first period. After quickly calling my mom to tell her the news, she congratulated me with so much excitement and enthusiasm that I thought she had lost her mind. *Why should I be excited about bleeding every month for the next 40 years!* While my sweet mom was trying to make it a positive experience (which I now appreciate), I couldn't help but dread everything having to do with periods and puberty.

My unpredictable body was taking me for a ride, and I was clueless about what was happening.

HELLO, HORMONES

A few months later, PMS came knocking. Her grand entrance was a little too obvious. First came the debilitating cramps that felt like someone was chopping up my insides and made me want to curl up in a ball and never leave my bed. Next came the excessively oily skin and hair, to the point that I was showering and shampooing my hair twice a day (which I now know only made it worse). That was followed by a long list of equally lousy symptoms like severe acne that lingered for months, dramatic mood swings that scared my parents, mild depression, cyclical weepiness, brain fog, cravings, painful bloating, constipation, severe breast tenderness, fatigue, and insomnia. The worst part was, as much as those symptoms sucked, I thought they were completely normal—and so did everyone around me. I was now a woman with a period, and this is what was supposed to happen. "It's just hormones," everyone said.

The problem is that hormones can make your life downright miserable if they aren't fluctuating within optimal ratios. Hormones control more than most people think; they act as the master switches for growth, reproduction, mood, metabolism, weight, energy, brain function, libido, and the appearance of your skin, hair, and nails. From a young age, women are fed an abundance of ideas about hormones. *PMS symptoms are normal. Most hormonal conditions are incurable. Hormonal chaos is "part of being a woman." The two options we have are to suck it up or take the birth control pill.*

The belief that hormones can only be tamed through medication is false, and these ideas are severely outdated. If we provided young girls with the tools, resources, and education to understand the ride of womanhood—fluctuating hormones and all—it would encourage a more positive connection to their bodies from the beginning. It would help eliminate the confusion, negativity, and sense of helplessness that I once felt, and so many young women feel, as their bodies start—and continue—to change.

Sure enough, by age 16, I had had enough and asked my mom if I could go on the pill—mostly because I yearned for clear, beautiful skin, and a life without cramps. It felt like my oily, acne-ridden and makeup-covered face was all anybody could see, which sucked my confidence dry. I've blogged about my journey with acne numerous times, but my biggest insecurity was always my skin. I would marvel at any girl with clear, radiant skin and wonder what on earth I was doing wrong. Since many of the girls in my high school were already on the pill for their periods and skin (and probably for other reasons, too), I wanted to join the club. Easier periods, clear skin, and pregnancy prevention? Um, yes, please! Going on

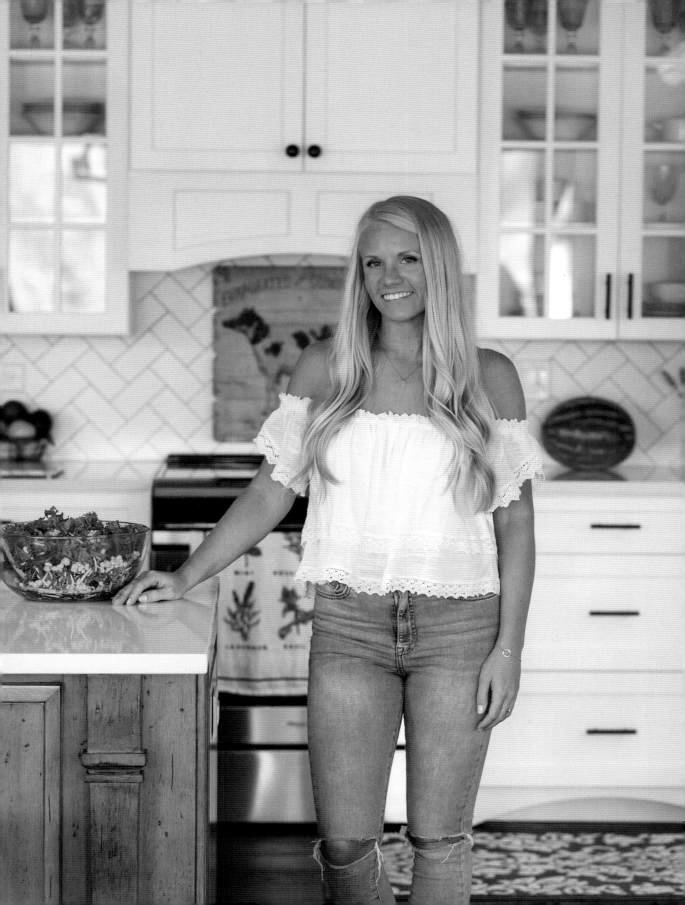

the pill couldn't have been easier. While many of my symptoms lessened while on the pill (we will get into why and how this happens in chapter three), my skin was still acting out. A dermatologist prescribed six months of a harsh medication that was popular at the time.

GOING VEGAN

The medication cleared up my skin fairly well for the rest of high school and throughout college. At age 25, green juices sparked my interest in holistic health and nutrition, and I began to question everything I was putting in and on my body. Then, on a cold Friday night in February 2014, I had a life-changing experience while watching a documentary called *Vegucated*. In an hour, everything I thought I knew about our food system blew up in my face, and I was left standing at a crossroads. While sick to my stomach, tears and mascara running down my face, I decided to go vegan right then and there. I knew nothing about the lifestyle at the time, but it felt like the universe closed the door on my previous life, and I had to move forward as a vegan. I know what you're thinking. This girl is dramatic! But it felt right, and everything about the vegan lifestyle instantly resonated with me.

This major lifestyle change prompted the start of my vegan recipe and lifestyle blog, *The Glowing Fridge*. That April, my little creative corner of the internet was born. One year later, blogging turned into my full-time career.

I wrote this book to be inclusive of all women. You do not have to be vegan or plant-based to follow the Happy Hormone Method. I purely wanted to create a space where that is possible. You can thrive with happy hormones *and* be vegan or plant-based, as long as you take the right precautions (which I will address), stay on top of your health by getting a full blood and hormone panel done every six months, and make adjustments as necessary.

Note: I use the terms "'vegan" and "plant-based" interchangeably throughout the book. Technically, vegan refers to an animal-free lifestyle, while plant-based refers only to an animal-free way of eating.

Two months into my vegan journey, I quit the pill, and my skin went haywire—in the worst way possible. Just like that, I was back at square one and had acne as an adult. Eating whole plant foods helped to heal my skin as I eliminated many of the inflammatory foods I had been eating (like dairy and processed junk), but it remained far from clear. Deep down, I sensed my skin issues were hormone-related but felt lost as to what steps to take to heal from within. By age 27, two years into my vegan journey, I had lost all hope for ever having clear skin or a regular period without severe PMS symptoms.

DISCOVERING *THE WOMANCODE*

At one point, a book on hormone health called *WomanCode,* written by Alisa Vitti, started popping up on blogs I was following and in my social media feeds. I took it as a sign and ordered the book. After reading the first chapter, a new fire ignited inside my soul.

From that moment on, all aspects of my life shifted again. How I approached PMS symptoms, how I cared for myself and my emotional health, how I ate and exercised, as well as my social life and my focus on my blogging career. I had a newfound sense of purpose, and a drive to learn everything I possibly could about hormone health and how to balance them naturally, without medication.

WomanCode acted as a handbook for many of my hormone-related issues and laid the foundation for my knowledge of hormones. Alisa is one of the reasons I'm writing this book. She taught me that every single PMS symptom I've ever dealt with is not normal and should not be expected, but instead taken as an indication of an internal imbalance. She taught me how to balance my blood sugar and eat cyclically to nourish my fluctuating endocrine system. She taught me that my body does not just have one setting like that of a man's, but rather many settings that are constantly moving through the four phases of my monthly menstrual cycle. She even taught me that doing intense cardio exercise in the second half of my cycle can actually increase my chances of weight gain. Her greatest gift was providing me with the permission I needed to pay special attention to my body instead of writing it off as broken as I had done for most of my life.

For me, Alisa normalized what being a woman is all about. I learned to accept and embrace my period, which was the opposite of what I used to do. I learned never to feel ashamed for talking about periods or blood or cervical mucus or anything that society labels as "taboo" or "gross" because all of these things are normal, healthy experiences for *every woman*. They are far from gross, and it's about time to empower and educate women by talking about periods and hormone health more openly.

I began studying hormone function and the very complex endocrine system (although the learning process never ends). From there, I experimented with different eating and lifestyle programs for my fluctuating hormones, while staying true to my plant-based vegan lifestyle. This became the most challenging part, as most programs included animal foods. My goal was to create a community and plan that would accommodate women who follow a vegan or plant-based lifestyle and are *also* interested in balancing their hormones naturally. Over time, my very own accessible program for living with happy hormones was born.

EXPERIENCING HAPPY HORMONES

I experienced noticeable improvements as early as the second month of my program with less cramping, bloating, and acne, as well as an increase in energy and motivation. My cycle started to balance out, going from 42 days down to a normal length of 28–30 days. I started sleeping better and felt less moody and depressed in my luteal phase (also known as the PMS phase, more on that in chapter 12). After six months, I felt incredible but was still experiencing breakouts along my jawline. It wasn't until I quit sugar and worked on my gut health that my hormonal acne completely disappeared for good.

Now that I know the ins and outs of my cycle, what is normal for my body, and have experienced how amazing life can be on the other side, I want to help others feel the same way.

Living with balanced hormones provides a powerful and deep connection to your body.

In this book, I'll teach you about the endocrine system and how to leverage its predictable functionality with your life each month, while syncing it with your career, social life, sex, food, workouts, beauty regimens and more. I'll also teach you how stress affects hormonal balance and share different ways to manage real-life stressors, along with why ovulation is the most important part of your menstrual cycle, how to identify different types of cervical mucus to track ovulation and how to promote ovulation. You'll learn how to view your period blood as your internal health report card, bring your period back if it's gone missing, and make the bleeding phase of your cycle more enjoyable.

You will discover why PMS symptoms happen and how to prevent them or eliminate them with food, herbs, and supplementation. Find out which nutrients, vitamins, and minerals are imperative for hormone balance, and which cycle phase to eat them. Not only will this book help you gain a deeper understanding of your menstrual cycle and fertility, but it will also amplify an intuitive connection with your body that lives within you, just waiting to be discovered.

Hormone imbalances don't happen overnight; they come from your daily choices.

A SETBACK

In April of 2018, right around the time I started writing this book, I intuitively knew something was wrong. I began to feel like I couldn't get out of bed in the mornings and my mind turned into a very dark, depressing place that made it hard to concentrate or feel happy. I got my hormones tested and found myself on the verge of hypothyroidism due to hypothalamic-pituitary axis dysregulation (also known as HPA-axis dysregulation or "adrenal fatigue," which you'll learn about in chapter 1), on top of low progesterone levels.

I knew it was my endocrine system's way of responding to too many life changes and too much stress. I brought my hormone lab results to a gynecologist, and her response was very disheartening. Regarding my low progesterone levels, she told me that I only need progesterone if I'm trying to get pregnant. Immediately I knew we were on different planets. That's like telling a man he only needs testosterone when he's trying to get a woman pregnant. Men would never accept that answer, so why should women? The fact that the gynecologist believed women's hormones are only useful for making babies represents a sad misconception in our culture (and is an issue I could write a whole other book about). She didn't even think to test my nutrient levels, find a possible underlying cause of my low progesterone, or ask me any relevant questions about my overall health.

After that, I decided to meet with a naturopath who spoke the same language and looked to treat my body as a whole. Sure enough, she found that my vitamin D levels were low, and my cortisol levels were out of whack, both of which affected my HPA-axis and hormone production. We came up with a plan consisting of new stress management skills, a better sleep routine, meditation, reduced caffeine intake, and new supplementation, as well as adding more sea vegetables to my diet (like kelp and dulse because they contain high amounts of iodine) and adding sea salt to my lemon water to help replenish lost mineral stores. In a couple of months, I was feeling better than ever.

The point of sharing this experience is to show you that the Happy Hormone Method can't outwork a stressful lifestyle. Following this program may force you to hone in on the hard stuff and go against the way you've always done things. But that's the beauty of it—and how you bring about change. Whether it's your addiction to working too much, pushing your body too hard at the gym, scheduling more than you can handle, staying in a toxic relationship, or whatever it may be, every stressor needs to be evaluated as part of this program. Of course, we will always have some amount of stress in our lives, but if you want to provide a strong foundation for your body to achieve optimal hormonal health, it's important to establish new ways of coping with stress. If you find this is too difficult to manage on your own, I highly recommend talking to a therapist or mental health professional or meeting with a naturopath to help navigate you through the initial steps. They can provide powerful tools and resources, so you don't have to wade through difficult or stressful situations alone.

THE POWER OF DAILY CHOICES

Although this experience was frightening, disheartening, and made me question everything, I archived it as a wake-up call that my body can only handle so much at one time. I was reminded once again that this is an all-encompassing lifestyle. I had to dig deeper and make some big changes to my attitude, sleep, caffeine consumption, workouts (I had to stop doing intense gym workouts and switch to a home routine using bodyweight training, resistance bands, and ankle weights) and how I handle day-to-day stress. The body works synergistically. One night of inadequate sleep can affect your eating habits, which can create imbalanced blood sugar levels that can spiral into a week of eating junk or drinking too much alcohol and throw off your menstrual cycle and ovulation. Every system in your body works together.

The sooner you can wrap your mind around the huge impact your daily choices have on your endocrine system and fertility as a whole, the better off you will be. So, while this program may not be a quick overnight fix, it is a lifestyle that keeps on giving at every stage of your life. The longer you stick with it, the bigger the payoff, especially during times of major hormonal shifts (like pregnancy and perimenopause).

FIND YOUR "WHY"

Think about your goals for your present self and future self. Whether your goal is to feel more connected, open the lines of communication with your inner guidance system, balance your hormones for future fertility, feel better overall and more like yourself, find your cyclical rhythm, lose weight, clear up your skin, or follow a unique female-focused monthly routine, it's all about what matters to *you*. To get the most out of this book, you must find your *why*.

My ultimate goals were to have clear skin throughout the whole month and abolish all PMS symptoms (which I achieved). In the first couple of months, all I could handle was adding in a few of the recommended foods because, at the time, I was very set in my routine ways of eating and exercising. Each cycle phase felt unfamiliar and new (except for the menstrual phase, of course). As I kept with it and introduced new aspects of the program while tracking my fluctuating signs and symptoms, each cycle phase started to feel more familiar and empowering.

It takes time to wrap your head around hormone health and education. Learning is ongoing. But now I can look back and see how far I've come, the immense body knowledge I've gained and how connected I feel, and that is the ultimate gift that I wish to give you.

Depending on your relationship with your cycle, you may feel most comfortable starting small and familiarizing yourself with the phases in chapters 9 through 12 before doing a complete lifestyle overhaul. You can incorporate as much or as little of this program into your life as you desire. Start slowly by changing or adding one thing per month, or dive in head first. There are no rules and adjusting your mindset to focus on the long-term benefit will take off the pressure and relieve any overwhelming feelings. There is no harm in following only one part, some parts or all parts of this program because only good can come from it. But keep in mind, the sooner you incorporate aspects of the Happy Hormone Method the quicker you will see results and feel better.

It's worth mentioning that sometimes I fall off the wagon and eat out more than I should, or drink too much on a weekend and find myself in a slump. Life happens, vacations happen, celebrations happen, and stress happens. Don't be hard on yourself. Get right back on track when you can with the next meal, work-out, or meditation. It's such a comfort to know that living with happy hormones is always within reach.

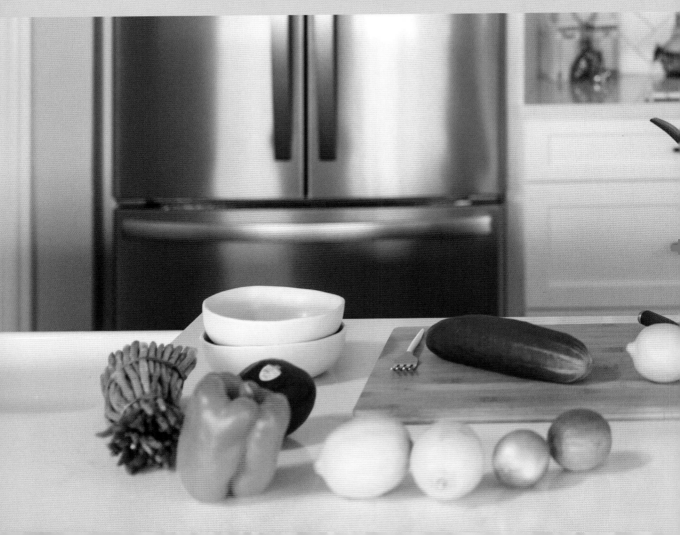

REDISCOVERING YOUR BODY

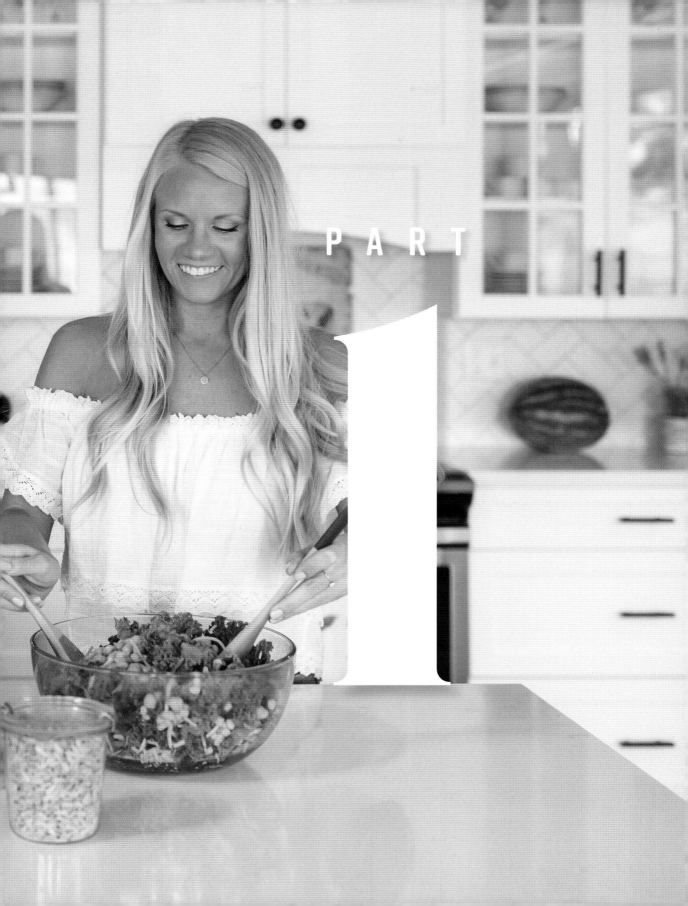

PART

1

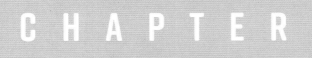

CHAPTER

1

YOUR ENDOCRINE SYSTEM

THE FIRST STEP TOWARD HAPPY HORMONES IS to develop a basic comprehension of what your endocrine system is, how it works, what disrupts it and how it strives for balance by using its natural intelligence. Having some understanding of hormone function is imperative for knowing your fluctuations and how to leverage them. This will help you optimize your endocrine system as a whole, through daily choices.

Your endocrine system is beautifully complex and strong. It's made up of glands that communicate with each other. Each gland secretes hormones to regulate specific bodily functions and behavior. The glands are either triggered by internal events such as ovulation or menstruation, external events like running from danger, extremely stressful situations, or other things like medication, toxins, or poor diet. The system is comprised of the pituitary gland, pineal gland, thyroid gland, parathyroid glands, adrenal glands, pancreas, ovaries (females), and testicles (males).

Hormones are chemical messengers that are constantly striving to keep balance in your body by helping regulate growth and development, metabolism, appetite, digestion, sleep cycles, reproductive functions, stress response, and mood. They have endless responsibilities. Without hormones, you wouldn't grow to reach the stages of life such as puberty, menstruation, pregnancy, or menopause. You wouldn't be able to produce breast milk for your newborn or metabolize food for energy. Hormones influence your hunger levels, heart rate, temperature, weight, skin, hair growth, brain function, mood, libido, energy levels, stress levels, sleep quality, immunity, ovulation, and menstruation.

As you will learn throughout this book, your hormones aren't only dictating your period— they're running the show.

Common Signs and Symptoms of Hormone Imbalance

- **SKIN, HAIR AND BODY:** acne, oily skin, dry skin, dullness, eczema, skin rashes, hair loss, thinning hair, extra hair on upper lip or chin, dandruff, brittle or breaking nails, excessive sweating, sweaty palms, night sweats, hot flashes, changes in sensitivity to heat and cold, blurred vision, vaginal dryness, early or late puberty

- **DIGESTION AND ELIMINATION PATHWAYS:** bloating, constipation, diarrhea, loose stools, irritable bowel syndrome, water retention, weight gain, going to the bathroom more or less than usual, inflammation, body odor, puffiness

- **PMS AND MENSTRUAL CYCLE:** cramps, breast tenderness/swelling, fibrocystic breasts, premenstrual spotting, irregular periods, painful periods, heavy periods, missing periods, late periods, anovulation, mood swings, irritability, depression, cyclical migraines, unexplained infertility, fatigue, mental fog, weepiness, fibroids, ovarian cysts, Polycystic Ovarian Syndrome, endometriosis

- **STRESS AND METABOLISM:** hypothyroidism, metabolic syndrome, diabetes, cravings (carbs, sugar, and chocolate), weight gain, caffeine dependency, insomnia, waking up in the middle of the night, anxiety, low libido

HOW PMS SYMPTOMS START

Your endocrine system is strong yet sensitive, so being exposed to daily endocrine-disrupting toxins (which you'll learn about in chapter 2), a poor diet, poor gut health, blood sugar imbalances, and the stress of day-to-day life can throw off hormone ratios. Hormones thrive on teamwork to keep your ratios within optimal ranges. If one hormone is out of range, the other hormones are affected too, thus creating symptoms like cramps, bloating, hormonal acne, cyclical depression, sadness for no reason, breast tenderness, mood swings, and fatigue. These are your body's attempt to alert you to this lack of balance, but we often write our symptoms off as expected or normal. It's okay to experience mild symptoms occasionally, but if they appear every month and remain unresolved for an extended period, they can lead to severe depression or a chronic hormonal condition like

PCOS, endometriosis, or hypothyroidism. You may get to this point and suddenly feel like your body has failed you, but the reality is, you've had many clues (symptoms) over time, and you didn't know how to address them. This is likely because a) you weren't taught how or b) you've been given incorrect information and led to believe medication is the only way these symptoms can be fixed.

PMS-related symptoms do not reflect healthy menstrual cycles and should not be expected every month. They are a cry for help as your body tries to restore balance. Depending on your lifestyle, genetic factors and how long these conditions go unanswered, they can lead to obesity, hypertension, diabetes, heart disease, cancers, premature aging, infertility, hysterectomies, and other conditions. This is why I focus on tracking your symptoms throughout your cycle and to understand the long-term impact of daily choices.

Did you know . . .

In 2016, the U.S. fertility rate fell to the lowest reproduction numbers since the CDC started keeping records back in 1909. An estimated 20 million Americans have some form of thyroid disease, and up to 60 percent of them are unaware of their condition. In the U.S., Polycystic Ovarian Syndrome (PCOS) affects one in every ten women of childbearing age, fibroids occur in three out of every ten women, and one in ten women has endometriosis. An estimated 12 million American women experience clinical depression each year. For U.S. women of reproductive age, hysterectomies are the second most frequently performed surgical procedure—after cesarean sections.

While I'm not trying to scare you, I share these statistics to show that women's bodies are crying for help. We must look for alternative ways to bring them back into balance, which is what *The Happy Hormone Guide* is all about.

THE HPA AXIS

The HPA axis (also known as the hypothalamic pituitary adrenal axis) is a complex communication network between the hypothalamus, pituitary, and adrenal glands that intertwine the endocrine and central nervous systems. These three glands work together to govern your stress response (fight or flight) as well as your emotions, metabolism, digestion, energy levels, libido, and immunity, ultimately connecting the mind and body.

It all starts in the brain, with your hypothalamus. Think of your hypothalamus as the hormone control center: it gets input from everyone and decides when to release hormones (from the pituitary gland). Its job is to regulate emotional responses, sleep, body temperature, hunger, and thirst. The hypothalamus can decide to stop or delay ovulation or menstruation temporarily due to stress, gut problems, lack of sleep, excessive caffeine, trauma, exposure to toxins, and more. Your hypothalamus thrives when you make healthy daily choices.

HOW STRESS AFFECTS YOUR BODY

During a stressful or threatening situation, the hypothalamus triggers an initial adrenaline rush resulting in a faster heartbeat, increased blood pressure and heightened alertness. Then, it signals your pituitary gland to release adrenocorticotropic hormone (ACTH), which prompts the adrenal glands to produce cortisol, your main fight-or-flight steroid hormone. Cortisol has a handful of jobs, but its main job is to manage blood sugar levels by increasing glucose (energy) and delivering it to your brain and muscles during threatening situations or exercise. It also acts as a natural alarm system to help your body wake up in the morning, fights off infection, and promotes tissue breakdown. Anytime there is an inflammatory response in the body, a release of cortisol can be expected. This means it's important to reduce or eliminate inflammatory foods like gluten, dairy, and refined sugar (more on this in chapter 4).

Cortisol levels should be highest in the morning around 8 a.m. and taper off throughout the day so you can sleep soundly at night. We need cortisol in acute amounts, but not in the chronically high amounts that are often triggered by our modern, stressful world. Continuously high levels of cortisol can lead to weight gain (specifically, belly fat), depression, heart disease, digestive issues, sleep issues, anxiety, headaches, and impaired brain and memory function. Alternatively, you can wake up with low cortisol in the morning and feel depressed or extremely tired during the day, and then experience a cortisol surge at night, causing sleep troubles. Having low cortisol levels is your brain's way of removing inflammation by down-regulating hormone production to make you feel tired in the hopes that you will rest and give your body a chance to heal.

ADRENAL FUNCTION AND HPA AXIS DYSREGULATION

No bigger than the size of walnuts, your adrenal glands sit atop each kidney and depend on signals from the pituitary gland to keep your sympathetic nervous system switched "on." As long as the brain continues to perceive something as dangerous or stressful, the adrenals are continuously signaled to produce cortisol and adrenaline. Whether these stressors are life-threatening or not, the adrenal glands are signaled to respond the same, no matter what the circumstance.

This brings us to adrenal fatigue. The modern, medically-accepted term for adrenal fatigue is HPA Axis Dysregulation, and it refers to changes in cortisol levels—either having too much or too little. This can wreak havoc on the HPA axis and related hormones, eventually leading to an altered stress response as the body becomes desensitized to the constant release of stress hormones, which can lead to total burnout or system breakdown (as well as excessive bone or muscle loss, high blood sugar, and insulin resistance). When any one part in the HPA axis is not running smoothly, it affects the next series of reactions and so on. For example, if you have chronically elevated cortisol levels, your hypothalamus may decide it's not the best time to reproduce because you are too stressed out. This means it can temporarily stop ovulation which inherently affects progesterone levels, and then affects your period by causing it to temporarily disappear or become irregular, not to mention the addition of PMS symptoms that come with low progesterone and/ or anovulation (lack of ovulation).

Dysregulation is essentially a communication break down or halt between all parts of the HPA Axis due to chronic activation of the stress response. It is your body's way of protecting you, in the hopes that you will slow down and rest. In turn, your brain dials back on the stimulation it sends from the pituitary to the adrenals, causing the adrenal glands to slow the production of cortisol and adrenaline. This is how the term "adrenal fatigue" came to be. The term is still used (it is used throughout this book) but can be a bit misleading because adrenal glands do not retire, get "fatigued," or give out the way the ovaries can. Thus, "adrenal fatigue" is not recognized in conventional medicine as a medical condition (unless you have Addison's Disease or Cushing's Disease, which relate to adrenal gland dysfunction).

The symptoms of HPA Axis Dysregulation are real and often accompanied by extremely low energy (no matter how much sleep you get), severe brain fog, depression, anxiety, little motivation, poor immunity, and dependence on caffeine. It's as if you are constantly functioning with a low battery. HPA Axis Dysregulation is a strong message to take stress-reducing protocols seriously. Otherwise, the body will never have a chance to repair so you can feel better and have natural energy again.

Your body functions by switching between the sympathetic nervous system (fight or flight) and parasympathetic nervous system (rest and digest). Internal healing and repair are done in the parasympathetic nervous system, which focuses on a "rest and digest" response to calm your body down after stress or trauma has subsided. As you can imagine, always hovering in "on" mode and unable to find any sense of peace or security can majorly affect the body as it pushes non-essential tasks like digestion, reproduction (ovulation), and immunity to the side. It does this thinking they can be dealt with at a later, less stressful time but unfortunately, that time doesn't come if you are constantly triggering cortisol.

How you respond to stress is unique to you and based on past experiences, genetics, and how well you care for your body. All you can do to bring the HPA Axis back into balance is alter your stress and relaxation approach, balance your blood sugar with each meal, tweak your diet and supplement regimen, and give the body time to heal (which can take 3–12 months, depending on the severity of the dysregulation). We will cover all of these things in future chapters. What's important to know now is that it's imperative to begin practicing a stress-reducing self-care routine. There are a variety of relaxation exercises that can help regulate cortisol levels and HPA Axis communication and switch your body into the parasympathetic "healing" mode.

HPA-AXIS HEALING ACTIVITIES

- ☐ Meditation and mindfulness
- ☐ Vagal exercises (look them up) to turn on the "rest and digest" response
- ☐ Neurofeedback
- ☐ Acupuncture
- ☐ Massage
- ☐ Reading
- ☐ Spending time in nature
- ☐ Spending time with people you love
- ☐ Brisk walking or light exercise to get the blood flowing
- ☐ Yoga inversion poses
- ☐ Bodyweight training
- ☐ Journaling
- ☐ Practicing gratitude
- ☐ Epsom salt baths
- ☐ Relaxing when you're tired instead of pushing through
- ☐ Positive self-talk
- ☐ Seeking counsel for emotional trauma or past experiences
- ☐ Deep breathing exercises
- ☐ Regular orgasms (!)
- ☐ Laughing
- ☐ Doing more of what you love
- ☐ Reducing caffeine and alcohol
- ☐ Eliminating sugar and processed foods
- ☐ Establishing regular meal times
- ☐ Having a regular sleep routine
- ☐ Focusing on the joys of life

Note: Refer to my supplement recommendations and treatment options for Stress and HPA Axis Healing as well as Brain Support on page 91.

SLEEP FOR HORMONE BALANCE

We know that proper sleep and rest is critical. We hear this constantly, so why don't we listen? Some of us get so caught up in the daily grind that we miss out on quality sleep and don't think much about the consequences. Sleep when you die, right? In our culture, it's almost as if adequate sleep is looked down upon as a waste of time. You may receive praise for sleeping less and achieving more, but that mindset is very backward and troubling for hormone balance and will most definitely catch up with you. Sleep deprivation can cause depressive-like effects, anxiety, and increased stress because it's more difficult to be productive when you don't get a good night's sleep, not to mention the cravings for sugar and carbs due to a lack of energy. None of this supports hormonal balance.

Sleep does wonders for your body. While sleeping, your body is actively repairing and recovering from the day. Cortisol levels and HPA-axis stabilize, energy levels are restored, tissue growth and repair occurs, appetite hormones are regulated, melatonin—a very potent antioxidant and sleep hormone that reduces inflammation—is released, human growth hormone (which deep cleans your cells while you sleep) is released, and insulin sensitivity is improved. If your sleep is cut short, you miss out on all of these amazing restorative activities that help you feel refreshed and energized in the morning. Consider proper sleep as one of the most important elements in balancing your hormones.

I'm not the biggest fan of saying you must get a certain number of hours of sleep, but the optimal amount is generally considered to be 7-8 hours of continuous, restorative sleep, and you wake up feeling well-rested. Also, know that sleep quality can vary throughout your cycle—for instance, you may experience PMS-related insomnia during your luteal phase due to the fluctuations of estrogen in relation to progesterone, especially if the ratio is not optimal. This is why a sleep routine is highly beneficial.

YOUR SLEEP ROUTINE

What do you watch before bed? Does it make your heart race? Does it trigger cortisol? Does it give you anxiety or nightmares? Do you consume caffeine too late in the day, or sugary, late-night snacks? Do you rely on alcohol to unwind? Does a bright light shine through your window at night, or does a light from your alarm clock or cable box interrupt your shut-eye? Every single one of these factors can affect your sleep quality.

Consider relaxing activities before bed like taking an Epsom salt bath, reading, essential oils, drinking herbal tea or taking herbs to help with sleep. Also, I can't

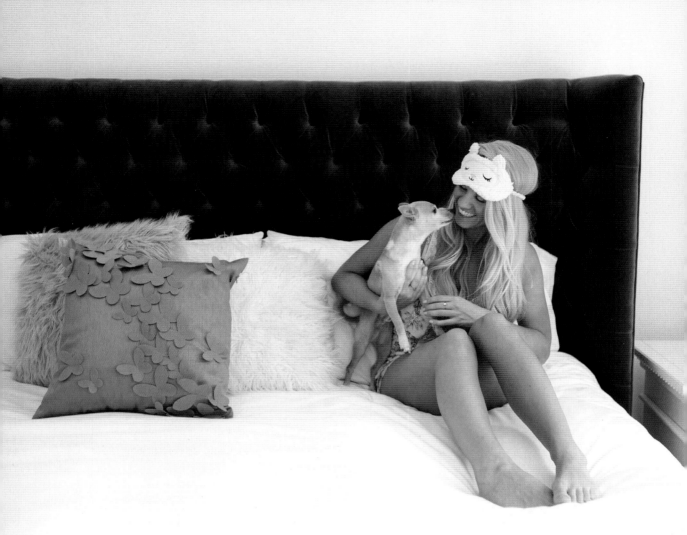

recommend magnesium glycinate enough, especially before bed, because it calms the nervous system, reduces anxiety, and primes your body for sleep. Since a cool, dark room creates an ideal environment for sleep, consider sleeping with an eye mask or using blackout shades. I put my phone on airplane mode every night to suspend interruptions and radio-frequency signals. I know in different stages of life sleep can seem downright impossible, especially if you are a new parent, but all you can do is try to rest as much as possible.

See supplements and herbal recommendations for sleep support and insomnia in the Herbs and Supplement section on page 90.

Exercising with HPA Axis Dysregulation

You want to feel good and energized after exercise. Pushing yourself while struggling with HPA Axis Dysregulation will only worsen your symptoms. You can still exercise in alignment with each cycle phase, but you'll want to modify exercises during the first half (follicular and ovulatory) and avoid high impact cardio, at least until your HPA Axis heals. Focus on walking, gentle yoga, or pilates. When I struggled with dysregulation, my favorite exercise was to stream p.volve™ videos and still is, to this day. They're low-impact, but you can feel the burn.

HORMONE IMBALANCE AND DEPRESSION

I want to touch on the mental and emotional aspect of not only HPA Axis Dysregulation, but hormone imbalance. When I was at my lowest point and extremely frustrated with being tired, lacking the brain power to concentrate and feeling deeply sad for no reason, my emotions brought out the worst in me. Because my progesterone, estrogen, and cortisol levels were so low, my mood was also very low. Little things would send me into a downward spiral, and I was always living on the verge of an emotional breakdown.

The weepiness and sadness factors of hormone imbalance are real. This is serious and can adversely affect your relationships, especially with your significant other, close family members, and friends. These people can be there to give emotional support but, as much as it sucks, they can't fix you or your hormones. I was self-sabotaging by starting unnecessary arguments, bringing up every little thing that annoyed me, and blaming my problems on everything and everyone but myself. I was incredibly sad and depressed but didn't realize it until I started healing and the dark clouds slowly lifted. Sometimes, when we are in the thick of sadness, we are unable to see the gravity of its effect on us and those around us.

I wanted to share my experience to show the link between hormone imbalance and depression. I don't think it's talked about enough, and many women are left in the dark when it comes to the root cause of their depression and anxiety.

At one point I considered antidepressant and anxiety medication but having the knowledge that my low mood was brought on by low hormone levels was enough motivation for me to choose a natural healing route. I'm not against medication because I know it is absolutely necessary for some people. But in my case, I knew that medication wouldn't address my underlying hormone imbalances or

HPA Axis Dysregulation and would only prolong my healing and create a reliance on medication.

If you are experiencing symptoms of depression, talk to your doctor and request to have a full blood and hormone panel done to see if it reveals an underlying hormone imbalance, nutrient deficiency or gut issue. If so, you'll clue into what's happening in your body that may be contributing to your sadness and anxiety. If you want to avoid using antidepressants or use them as a last resort but don't know where to start with natural healing, try the Happy Hormone Method for at least three months, and see if your symptoms subside or lessen.

Refer to my supplement recommendations and alternative treatment options for depression and anxiety on page 91.

THE ROLE OF YOUR THYROID

Menstrual problems are closely linked with thyroid conditions. Your thyroid is a butterfly-shaped gland located on the front of the throat. The largest of all the endocrine glands, it acts as your internal thermostat and master of metabolism by regulating body temperature, hunger, and energy expenditure. Out of the estimated 20 million Americans suffering from some type of thyroid disorder, more than half of them don't know their thyroid has been causing the hair loss, weight gain or inability to lose weight, mood imbalance, or depression.

The thyroid produces two main hormones, T3 (triiodothyronine) and T4 (thyroxine). These hormones stimulate calorie burn and metabolic processes like detoxification, digestion, and ovulation. They also influence mood regulation, cognitive function, sex drive, energy levels, sleep quality, and more. Undiagnosed thyroid disorders can majorly affect your life. The two most common disorders are hypothyroidism and hyperthyroidism.

SIGNS OF A SLUGGISH THYROID: HYPOTHYROIDISM

Hypothyroidism is the more common condition and signifies an underactive thyroid that's not producing enough thyroid hormones. Hypothyroid symptoms can include:

- ☐ Low basal metabolic rate which leads to unexplained weight gain or difficulty losing weight (even with a healthy diet and exercise)
- ☐ Puffy face or puffy eyes
- ☐ Eyelid twitching
- ☐ Dry skin (mostly on the scalp)
- ☐ Itching inside the ears
- ☐ Cracked heels

Signs of Sluggish Thyroid: Hypothyroidism continued...

- ☐ Cold feet and hands
- ☐ Hair loss or thinning hair
- ☐ Fatigue
- ☐ Depression
- ☐ Anxiety
- ☐ Brain fog
- ☐ Forgetfulness
- ☐ Sweaty palms
- ☐ Swollen neck
- ☐ Constipation
- ☐ Muscle weakness or stiffness
- ☐ Chronic headaches
- ☐ Slowed heart rate
- ☐ Exhaustion

High amounts of stress, iodine or zinc deficiency, and toxicity can also contribute to hypothyroidism.

SIGNS OF AN OVERACTIVE THYROID: HYPERTHYROIDISM

Hyperthyroidism is less common and refers to an overactive thyroid gland, producing too many thyroid hormones. This increases the body's metabolism and causes bodily functions to speed up. Symptoms include:

- ☐ Feelings of nervousness
- ☐ Anxiety
- ☐ Irritability
- ☐ Insomnia
- ☐ Extra bowel movements or diarrhea
- ☐ Racing heartbeat or heart palpitations
- ☐ Heat intolerance
- ☐ Excessive sweating
- ☐ Shortness of breath
- ☐ Dizziness
- ☐ Itching
- ☐ Hives
- ☐ Muscle weakness
- ☐ Bulging eyes
- ☐ Unexplained or sudden weight loss
- ☐ Fatigue
- ☐ Appetite change
- ☐ Vision change
- ☐ Thin or brittle hair

Graves disease, taking too many tablets of the T4 hormone, or having lumps on the thyroid can all contribute to hyperthyroidism.

Thyroid conditions often involve menstrual cycle problems as well, like heavy or light menstrual bleeding, miscarriage, postpartum depression, multiple periods per month, anovulatory cycles, and hypersensitivity to hormonal shifts throughout your cycle.

Natural Thyroid Support and Treatment

The following are treatment methods to support, correct, and rebalance your thyroid naturally. It's important to note that a comprehensive approach is necessary—it's not enough to take a supplement and hope it cures your thyroid condition. This type of natural support involves looking at your body as a whole.

- While often overlooked, there are several nutrients necessary for proper thyroid function, including zinc, iodine, selenium, and vitamins D and B. Make sure you are getting plenty of these nutrients

- Address gut health and gut problems like malabsorption of nutrients, unhealthy gut bacteria, and leaky gut, parasites, or infection

- Add probiotics and digestive enzymes into your diet

- Raw cruciferous vegetables can inhibit thyroid function, so always cook or lightly steam your Brussels sprouts, cauliflower, broccoli, kale, etc.

- Manage stress

- Get quality sleep

- Only drink filtered water to avoid chlorine, fluoride, and other chemicals in unfiltered tap water (and use a fluoride-free toothpaste)

- Eat foods rich in zinc (and copper, for counterbalance) like sesame seeds, pumpkin seeds, cashews, soybeans (edamame), sunflower seeds, tempeh, garbanzo beans, lentils, lima beans, and oats

- Switch to a gluten-free diet

- Avoid processed foods

- Eat more sea vegetables (kelp, dulse, and nori), which are natural sources of iodine

- Reduce the use of toxic, endocrine-disrupting products (see chapter 2)

- Consider working with a functional medicine doctor to find the root cause of your thyroid imbalance

If you're curious about having your thyroid tested, ask your doctor to do a comprehensive thyroid panel that includes TSH, Free and Total T4, Free and Total T3, Reverse T3, thyroid antibodies, TPO Ab, and Thyroglobulin Ab (to rule out autoimmune thyroid problems).

See more for thyroid support in the Herbs and Supplement section on page 89.

HORMONE TESTING

The only way to truly know what is going on with your hormones is to have your levels tested. However, you want to make sure they are being tested accurately and optimally before your doctor determines you are "normal" when you don't quite feel right. These labs are important because they will provide a baseline assessment and comparison for the future. Looking up symptoms, blindly guessing, and making your own protocol is not recommended (symptoms often appear similar for different imbalances, conditions, or deficiencies), and you may end up wasting money on unnecessary supplements that could worsen your hormone health or prolong the healing process.

There are a few different ways to go about testing. Traditionally, hormone testing is done via a serum (blood) test but, these days, we can use a serum (blood) or dried blood spot (for at-home testing), saliva, dried urine, or a combination of all three to get the full picture. You'll want to take an additional test in three months to track progress, and every 6–12 months after.

SERUM (BLOOD) TESTING: This is the most widely accepted and accessible way to test hormones in the conventional medical world, through your gynecologist or primary care practitioner. Serum is accurate for testing peptide hormones (like FSH, LH, prolactin, insulin, and thyroid hormones) as well as the sex hormone binding globulin (SHBG) and nutrient markers, but it's not good at predicting the bioavailability of sex hormones or providing a full picture of cortisol throughout the day. This is because serum tests only provide the total hormone levels circulating in your blood at that one moment, rather than the free (active) levels. This may cause your results to appear "normal" when in reality the majority of your hormones may be bound and therefore, inactive. It also becomes problematic because your hormone levels fluctuate throughout the month and it's ideal to have a comprehensive overview of every hormone ratio throughout your monthly cycle. Testosterone is an exception, as it can be tested in both total and free forms, providing a full picture.

DRIED BLOOD SPOT TESTING: This is an at-home form of collection where you prick your finger and place blood drops on a filter card. Once dry, blood spot cards are stable for shipment and storage. The dried blood format equates to serum blood testing. Its advantage over serum is that it eliminates the need for a complete blood draw and can be done from the comfort of your home.

SALIVA TESTING: This is a non-invasive form of testing that's accessible for at-home testing or naturopath patients. While it's hard to spit that much saliva into a plastic tube, it's great for those who are scared of needles or blood. It can also provide more accurate cortisol readings, as serum testing can reflect falsely high cortisol if patients are afraid. Since saliva is easier to collect, this form of testing provides multiple snapshots in time to see the bigger picture for specific symptoms of hormone excess or deficiency. For example, cortisol can be measured multiple times per day (morning, noon, afternoon, and night) and sex hormones can be measured throughout the month rather than just at one moment in time. Saliva testing is valuable because it looks at the free (active) levels thereby allowing us to see the availability of hormones at the cellular level, but it won't provide complete levels.

DRIED URINE TESTING (THE DUTCH TEST): DUTCH stands for Dried Urine Test for Comprehensive Hormones. It's an advanced assessment form of hormone testing that uses urine samples on filter card collection strips. It is the gold standard way of measuring adrenal, sex steroid hormone by-products and their respective metabolic pathways. By gauging how your body metabolizes hormones, it reveals the *types* of estrogen you are making, which shows how at-risk you are for certain estrogen-dependent cancers such as breast, ovarian, and uterine. Additionally, it's the most common method for testing brain neurotransmitters. What makes this test stand out from the blood tests ordered by your doctor or the saliva test from your naturopath is this: *every piece of* information you collect from other forms of testing can be collected with a single DUTCH test.

Because it is a more in-depth assessment, I recommend finding an expert (like a naturopath or functional medicine practitioner) who can understand and interpret the results and determine the next steps for treatment. While a conventional doctor may be able to understand your results, they most likely will not know how best to help you using alternative treatment methods.

Not every woman needs to take this advanced form of testing, especially if you are only experiencing mild symptoms. But for the woman who is very symptomatic, has already had blood or saliva testing done and still doesn't have answers, has a hormonal condition (like PCOS or endometriosis), is having trouble getting pregnant, or simply wants a complete, in-depth look into how her body is functioning, then the DUTCH test would be the best way to get specific answers.

For other women who have mild symptoms but want to check in with their body, I recommend doing a combined serum and saliva test through your doctor or naturopath or doing an at-home testing kit.

Note: If you are on hormonal birth control, then hormone testing results will be inaccurate. Wait three months after stopping birth control to start any testing.

Home Testing Kits

These tests can be ordered online or through a practitioner and done at home (always search online for coupon codes before buying tests), but a doctor or naturopath should review your results. Why do at-home testing? Unless your doctor thinks there is something wrong, they can't order a standard hormone test and bill your insurance. At-home testing is one way around that.

- **DUTCH DRIED URINE TEST:** See above (dutchtest.com)

- **FLOLIVING WOMEN'S HEALTH TESTING KIT THROUGH EVERLYWELL:** This easy testing kit uses dried blood spots and saliva collections throughout your cycle. Results are available within days via an online dashboard. FloLiving offers a 30-minute follow-up phone consultation. You can also print your results and present them to your doctor or naturopath (everlywell.com).

- **ZRT LABORATORY:** This lab provides numerous home testing kits using dried blood spot, saliva, or a combination for hormone balance, but they must be ordered through a practitioner. Providers can be found on their website (zrtlab.com).

NATUROPATHIC DOCTORS

I recommend meeting with a gynecologist or naturopathic doctor who is willing to explore natural solutions using a whole-body approach. Sometimes, it takes meeting with a few medical professionals and expanding your team to find the answers you want and need. Getting a second or third opinion never hurts, especially if you feel uncomfortable with your doctor's recommendations. Use the American Association of Naturopathic Physicians website to find a naturopath near you (naturopathic.org).

LAB TESTS WITH YOUR DOCTOR OR NATUROPATH

If you forego at-home tests and prefer to visit your doctor or naturopath, be sure to ask for the full hormone panel test that includes estrogen, progesterone, FSH and LH, as well as a full thyroid hormone panel, including TSH, T3, T4, and reverse T3. Most doctors will only want to test TSH, so make sure to ask for the full panel. If you have a 28-day cycle, it's best to have the tests taken on day three (for estrogen) and days 19–22 in the middle of your luteal phase (for progesterone).

You'll also want a complete blood panel. This will look at key nutrient biomarkers, anemia, red blood cell status, and more. The test can be done at any time of the month, and it will indicate any nutrient deficiencies you might have.

CHAPTER

2

TOXINS & DETOXIFICATION

WHILE CHATTING WITH A FRIEND ABOUT her new cleaning service for her home, she said their service was detailed and thorough, but she couldn't smell the "clean" smell when they were done. I pointed out that they might be using natural products because it's toxic for people to use chemicals all day. It made me think about how disconnected we are from natural smells, and how accustomed we've become to synthetic, toxic fumes on store shelves (just walking down that aisle gives me a headache).

I know that synthetic "clean" smell very well, and I used to think it made my space feel cleaner, too. What I didn't realize was how toxic this was to my endocrine system, and how detrimental it was to my hormone health (and most likely contributed to my acne).

ENDOCRINE-DISRUPTING CHEMICALS

Using toxic bleach and harsh cleaning products leaves a harmful, lingering residue for you, your family, and your pets. There are plenty of non-toxic ways to disinfect, clean, and freshen your home using natural ingredients. That way, you don't have to worry about breathing in toxic fumes, staining your clothes with bleach, or burning your hands from chemicals. Natural products are better for the environment, too.

Cleaning supplies aren't the only culprit when it comes to toxins. Before you walk out your front door in the morning, you're exposed to over a hundred endocrine-disrupting chemicals on average. These chemicals come from hand soap, laundry detergent, dryer sheets, hair products, body wash, body lotion, skin care, makeup, nail polish, deodorant, perfume, air fresheners, candles, scented sprays, cleaning products, and unfiltered tap water. Not to mention the chemicals used in dry cleaning services, lawn care services, salons and spas, building materials, farming, agricultural practices, the plastics in reusable containers and flame-retardants used on fabrics for furniture, rugs, and curtains. Most of these chemicals are not tested for their effects on human health because of how the U.S. regulates toxic chemicals.

You may be rolling your eyes because you've heard these chemicals are only harmful in high doses but *picture this:* you wake up and start getting ready for work. First, you brush your teeth with a conventional toothpaste made with triclosan and artificial sweeteners. You hop in the shower, and use body wash containing sulfates, parabens, and fragrance. You shampoo and condition your hair with more sulfates, parabens, and fragrance. Then you get out of the shower and apply a body lotion with polyethylene glycols (PEG's), mineral oil and fragrance, and roll on deodorant with aluminum, and then lather on face serums, moisturizers and makeup with more chemicals. Maybe you add some hair products and a spritz of perfume. Your body has just been overloaded with toxic substances before you even start your day, and this may happen several times per week. When you think about all of the environmental chemicals and pesticides in foods we encounter daily, it's no wonder our natural detoxification and elimination systems are overloaded.

These toxins may be fine in small amounts, but when you use them every single day, it becomes a much larger dosage. We now know that consistent low dose exposure in amounts thought to be acceptable are affecting hormone balance, and can also impact fertility and pregnancy.

HOW DO TOXINS AND CHEMICALS AFFECT HORMONE BALANCE?

Endocrine-disrupting chemicals (also known as EDC's) interfere with hormone action. They can mimic certain hormones to trick your system into over-producing some while under-producing others. They interfere with the proper elimination of estrogen in your body, which increases your risk for estrogen-dominant hormonal conditions such as PCOS and endometriosis. Some EDC's imitate estrogen—these are known as xenoestrogens. Xenoestrogens include bisphenol-a (BPA), parabens, phthalates, pesticides, and herbicides, to name a few.

If this feels overwhelming and alarming, it's because it is. It may sound like EDC's are unavoidable, but you can control a lot more than you think. It starts with the food and products you purchase. This isn't about being perfect but rather being aware and making the switch to non-toxic products and organic food whenever possible. The good news is, many companies and brands are catching on, listening to consumers and changing their formulas to become more "green" by including cleaner and safer ingredients.

Natural Beauty and Skincare Products

I'm a total beauty junkie and love experimenting with new products, but the following are my go-to brands ranging from skincare, makeup, haircare, and deodorant to nail polish, self-tanner, and sunscreen.

- **SKINCARE:** OSEA, Eminence Organics, Drunk Elephant, Herbivore Botanicals, Tata Harper, Marie Veronique, Pacifica, Acure, Juice Beauty
- **MAKEUP:** Lily Lolo (especially the big lash mascara), ILIA, Vapour, RMS, W3ll People, 100% Pure, Tarte, Fitglow Beauty, Cover FX
- **SHAMPOO & CONDITIONER:** Innersense, Acure, 100% Pure, Avalon Organics, Rahua
- **DRY SHAMPOO:** Kaia Naturals, Acure
- **BODY WASH:** Dr. Bronner's, Raw Sugar, or Shea Moisture
- **SUNSCREEN:** Supergoop!, Suntegrity 5-in-1 Tinted Moisturizing Sunscreen (for face)
- **DEODORANT:** Schmidt's, Native, Primal Pit Paste, Crystal deodorant
- **TOOTHPASTE:** Desert Essence, Tom's of Maine, Dr. Bronner's, Jason Natural
- **NAIL POLISH:** Zoya, Ella + Mila, Deborah Lippmann, Pacifica, JINSoon
- **NAIL POLISH REMOVER:** Zoya, Ella + Mila
- **SELF TANNER:** Vita Liberata, Eco Tan Face Tan Water, Tropic Sun Drops Gradual Tanning Serum, Chocolate Sun

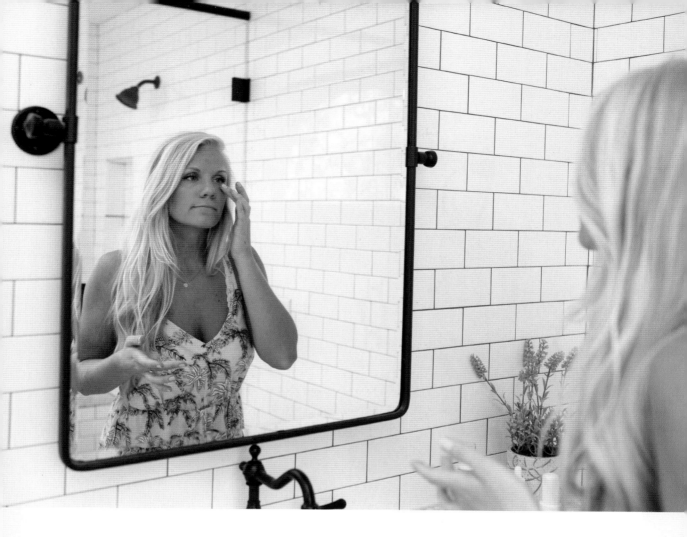

SYSTEMS OF DETOXIFICATION
AND ELIMINATION

Your body was designed to naturally detox through major elimination pathways including the liver, large intestine, kidneys, skin, and lymphatic system. Detoxification is your body's way of eliminating toxic waste. When these systems are working efficiently, you should feel great. But when your detoxification pathways are blocked, you end up with toxic buildup and a variety of unwanted symptoms. Luckily, there are plenty of things you can do to support your body's natural detox process, but first, let's go over how each system functions.

LIVER, LARGE INTESTINE, AND KIDNEYS

This two-phase process starts in the liver, where used-up hormones, digested food, medications, caffeine, toxins, and chemicals are filtered and metabolized. Your liver breaks down these substances from fat-soluble molecules into smaller, water-soluble molecules. One thing you must know is that this process is highly dependent on specific nutrients from the foods you eat. These nutrients include vitamins B and C, glutathione, selenium, and amino acids, which are stored in your liver for this very reason. If you aren't getting enough of these nutrients from your diet, your liver function will be impaired.

The second detoxification phase is crucial. As these substances are broken down into water-soluble molecules, they become free radicals making them more toxic than before. Therefore, they need to be moved out of the body as quickly as possible. These substances move through your gallbladder to combine with bile and move through the large intestine. This is where fiber comes into play. Ample amounts of fiber from your diet will bind to the waste in the large intestine to ensure a quick exit via a bowel movement. Now, if you are constipated, you run the risk of these toxic free radicals reabsorbing into the bloodstream through the large intestine, which is why adequate fiber and regular bowel movements are crucial.

Your kidneys are responsible for managing the volume and composition of fluids in the body, like regulating electrolyte balance (sodium, potassium, and calcium), maintaining balanced pH levels (acid-alkaline balance) and filtering blood. Located below your ribcage near the middle of your back, they also help regulate blood pressure, eliminate bacterial waste, and flush out extra water, which excretes from the bladder via urine.

See the Detox And Nourish Your Liver section on page 108 and the recommended Herbs and Supplements on page 89.

THE GUT-HORMONE CONNECTION

The synergistic connection between your gut microbiome and hormone health is incredible. The gut microbiome is made up of a complex community of bacteria, viruses, and microbes that do the work of digesting your food and synthesizing nutrients. In healthy adults, upwards of 100 trillion microbial cells are living in the gut, weighing in at approximately five pounds. The quality and diversity of their ecosystem dictate your health through brain function, digestion, metabolism, and hormone balance, and influence how you feel physically, mentally, and emotionally. It's not surprising that poor microbiome health is linked to depression, anxiety, cancer, blood sugar imbalances, and diabetes.

When hormonal symptoms are present, treating digestive health is crucial. Specifically, your microbiome affects hormone regulation and estrogen metabolism. In your gut lies a specific group of a bacteria called the estrobolome that produce an enzyme for metabolizing and clearing out used up estrogen. This means that poor gut health can result in estrogen-dominance with symptoms of heavy periods, bloating, acne, moodiness, painful cramps, low libido, infertility, PCOS, fibroids, and cysts. A continuous overload of estrogen can increase your risk for female cancers, hypertension, diabetes, and dementia.

Work on gut health and hormone health will follow. This means keeping your microbiome balanced by:

- Cutting out inflammatory foods like dairy, wheat, gluten, alcohol, sugar, processed foods, and vegetable oils (like canola, soybean, and corn oil)

- Providing it with plenty of micronutrients and ample fiber from fruits and vegetables

- Managing stress and cortisol levels

- Limiting caffeine

- Building up your good bacteria with probiotics

Happy Hormone Tip

Aim to chew each bite of food thoroughly before swallowing. This is an important part of the digestive process because it increases saliva production and signals to your stomach which enzymes to produce, while proactively helping to break down your food before it reaches your stomach. This takes practice, as most of us are in the habit of inhaling our food, which creates a lot of work for your digestive system and can cause bloating and abdominal pain. So, eat more slowly, chew your food, and take a moment to enjoy your meal.

YOUR SKIN

The next pathway of elimination is the largest organ of your body: your skin. Through sweating, your skin expels anything the liver and large intestine couldn't dispose of that's been stored in your tissues. Since your skin is the last stop for waste removal, many people experience skin symptoms when other elimination

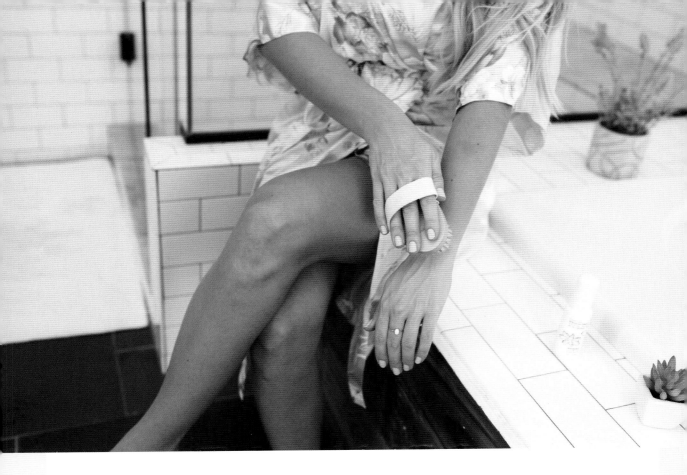

pathways aren't functioning properly, and there's a build up of toxins. These symptoms may include acne, eczema, rosacea, rashes, itching, and body odor. This is why you want to make sure what you are putting on your skin isn't making things even worse by clogging your pores or containing EDC's since your skin absorbs everything you apply on it.

THE LYMPHATIC SYSTEM

The primary function of your very complex lymphatic system is to transport lymph fluid made of infection-fighting white blood cells through a network of lymph nodes (you have about 600 of them), organs, and vessels. Think of it as a garbage truck driving along picking up waste, toxins, and excess fluid tucked away in your tissues and cells. The only problem is, nothing automatically pumps or moves the lymphatic system for you—it only pumps when you use your muscles. You'll notice a sluggish lymphatic system when you feel puffy (accumulation of extra fluid throughout the body and face) and have swollen feet or ankles. To prevent this, you want to make sure to incorporate regular activity and exercise into your lifestyle.

Your lymphatic system intricately connects to your immune system, so when lymph fluid is congested and stagnant, fluid can pool with the infectious bacteria, putting you at risk of getting sick, allergies, or sinus infections, and autoimmune conditions like lupus or rheumatoid arthritis. It's important to keep the lymph fluid flowing because some of your lymph nodes sit near sensitive areas such as your ovaries and breast tissue. Have you ever felt or noticed enlarged lymph nodes on your throat (tonsils), underarms, or groin area? These are your lymph nodes fighting off an infection or virus.

The only way to get lymph fluid flowing is through an activity like jumping or any vigorous movement. You can feel the lymph fluid draining in the back of your throat, which may make you want to swallow (don't worry, you can't taste it).

When the lymphatic system is regularly flowing, you are eliminating bacteria and getting rid of waste more quickly, which means you'll feel healthy and will be less likely to get sick.

LYMPHATIC DRAINAGE SUPPORTING ACTIVITIES

- [ ] Sweating to release toxins via exercise, infrared sauna, or steam room.

- [ ] Dry brushing to slough away dead skin cells and stimulate the movement of lymph fluid. Dry brushing supports your immune system and encourages natural detoxification (do it first thing in the morning to wake up, as it is super energizing).

- [ ] Alternating the water at the end of a shower from hot to cold a few times, to flush extra fluids and toxins from your skin cells as they contract and expand

- [ ] Take Epsom salt baths

- [ ] Get a lymphatic massage

- [ ] Rebounding (jumping on a mini trampoline)

- [ ] Avoiding antiperspirant deodorant with aluminum

Natural Oral Hygiene Essentials

Oral health deserves more attention than it receives. Prioritizing oral care supports detoxification, encourages digestive power, strengthens immunity, enhances your sense of taste, and ensures that your teeth and gums remain intact and healthy. Aside from these reasons, I make time for my oral care routine because it makes me feel cleaner and healthier and prevents bad breath. Here are a few of my favorite natural techniques.

OIL PULLING: The concept of oil pulling is an Ayurvedic tradition used for thousands of years to clean and detoxify the teeth and gums. It's the act of swishing around oil in the mouth for 10-20 minutes (before drinking water or brushing your teeth) to improve gum health, with the added effect of whitening. Since oil is "sticky," it navigates around your mouth, up into pockets and tiny areas where a toothbrush can't reach. Think of it as a natural antimicrobial mouthwash, where it dissolves bacteria and pulls out toxins and food remnants. Coconut oil is my favorite for this, but any vegetable-based oil will work (sesame, sunflower, or olive). Just make sure they are raw, organic, and unrefined. Spit the oil, in the garbage, then floss and brush for a dazzling white smile and super fresh breath.

TONGUE SCRAPING: Did you know bad breath often stems from bacteria left on your tongue? I started this Ayurvedic practice of tongue scraping because it cleans toxins and bacteria from the tongue, removes the excess coating, enhances your sense of taste, and gently stimulates your internal organs. A coating on the tongue indicates the presence of toxins which interrupt proper digestion, and we know how that affects our hormones. There are many different kinds of tongue scrapers. I opt for a surgical-grade stainless steel version.

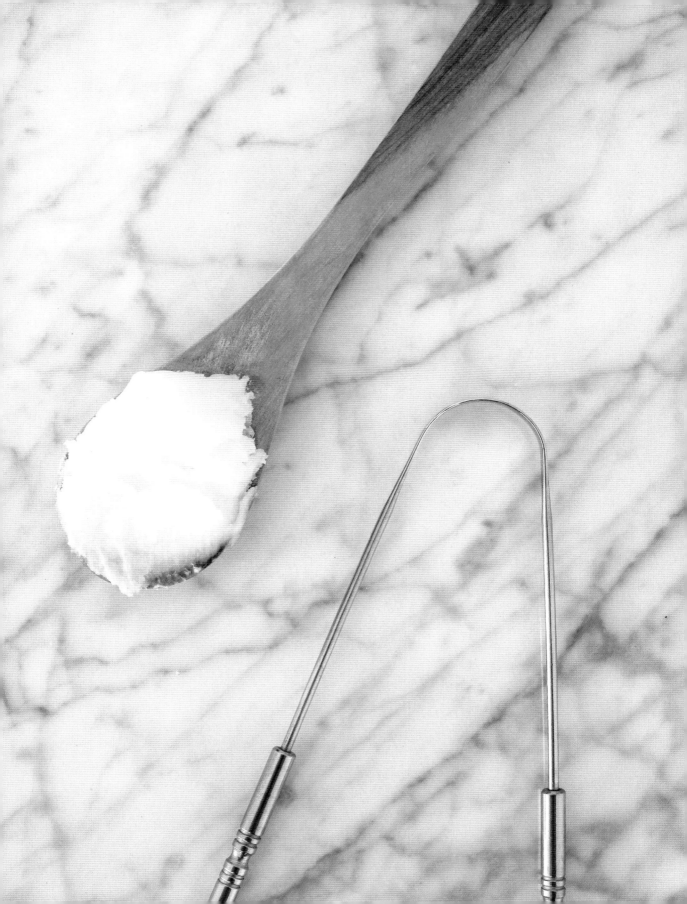

CHAPTER

3

BIRTH
CONTROL

WHILE THE BIRTH CONTROL PILL HAS BEEN revolutionary in providing women with the freedom of choice to prevent pregnancy, the reality is that most women are unaware of how the pill works, what systems it affects in the body, and the numerous risks and side effects that come along with it. While nearly 12 million women in the U.S. take birth control, the conversation about whether the risks outweigh the benefits remains a controversial one.

Hormonal birth control is not the path for me, but I won't judge. Some women prefer it. I believe women should have the freedom to decide for themselves—but *only* after knowing how hormonal birth control works, how it puts a band-aid on hormonal symptoms, the extensive side effects, as well as options for alternative methods. The issue is that most of this information is not conveyed to women before the pill is prescribed. I feel it's important to share what I've learned about birth control so that you can come to your decision from an informed place.

Please note that if you are on some form of hormonal birth control, then you will not experience the full benefits of the Happy Hormone Method because your natural hormonal fluctuations are turned off.

The early marketing ploys behind the birth control pill are unsettling. After it launched in the 1960s, women initially felt uneasy about taking the pill because at first, it made their periods disappear altogether. To combat their discontent, manufacturers of the pill added in a week of placebo sugar pills, so women would experience a pharmaceutically-induced bleed every 28 days and still feel like they were having a "natural" period (even though it's not a real period at all, just breakthrough bleeding).

This idea may sound harmless, but in reality, it is very misleading. The result is that the majority of women on the pill believe they are functioning naturally because they bleed every 28 days like clockwork when in actuality, their monthly bleed is pharmaceutically-controlled. The introduction of sugar pills resulted in women asking fewer questions and feeling less concerned about taking the pill, which instantly increased the pill's appeal and popularity—and revenue.

The pill works by *disrupting* the normal function of your endocrine system. By providing low doses of estrogen and progestin/progesterone, it interferes with communication between your brain and ovaries. This disrupts the HPA-axis (see page 24) and prevents ovulation (the release of an egg), thereby preventing pregnancy. The pill also prevents your body from producing fertile-quality cervical fluid which, as you will learn, is a healthy sign of fertility. Sperm can't live inside your vagina or travel anywhere near your egg without fertile mucus, so this also prevents pregnancy. Lastly, the pill stops your uterine lining (the lining that either houses an embryo or ends up being shed during menstruation) from fully developing. So, if an egg were to get fertilized somehow, it would have nowhere to implant, and you would not get pregnant. But all of these disruptions come at a cost.

Taking hormonal birth control shuts off ovulation, which in turn shuts off menstruation. As you will later learn, the event of ovulation is the only way your body can make progesterone, and adequate levels of progesterone are the only way to have a normal period. All of these components build on each other, which means ovulation is the most important part of your menstrual cycle. So, these beneficial hormones that naturally fluctuate through your body suppress when you take the pill. I know what you may be thinking: you don't want to get pregnant right now so who cares about ovulation or a real period? I get it because, at one point, I felt the same way. But the Happy Hormone Method is about optimizing each phase of your cycle to feel your best throughout the entire month—whether you want to get pregnant or not. To do that, you must fluctuate naturally through the four phases to truly harmonize your body.

Despite feeling disconnected from my body and not like myself, I stayed on the pill for ten years. In those ten years, not one medical professional relayed how the pill stops ovulation, menstruation, and natural cyclical changes. They failed to mention that it can deplete the body of key micronutrients (like vitamins B6 and B12, magnesium, folate, zinc, selenium, and vitamin E), which are essential to keep hormones in balance in the first place, or how it can alter and disturb your highly sensitive microbiome, which means taking a daily probiotic is necessary.

I was young and didn't care to know how the pill worked, but I also trusted that my doctor, who was filling my prescriptions month after month, would fill me in on necessary steps to improve my quality of life. Looking back, they all scooted me out the door as quickly as possible. If I ever brought up a negative side effect, they would recommend trying a different brand instead of getting to the root of my problem or symptom. They mentioned how the pill would "balance my hormones" (how ironic), clear up my skin (due to the synthetic estrogen stopping skin oil and sebum production), and eliminate cramps, which brings me to my next point.

SIDE EFFECTS OF HORMONAL BIRTH CONTROL

Oral contraception has evolved into this miracle cure for all the period symptoms we don't want to deal with because they admittedly suck. From acne to painful cramps, heavy periods to mood swings we hear, "just take this pill, and your symptoms will disappear." Often, the pill is used as a treatment to "normalize" periods more so than its intended purpose of contraception. Doctors love to prescribe the pill because it's an easy one-and-done prescription that acts as a temporary band-aid for period problems. This sends the message early on that the pill can control and regulate your cycle with hormones which are superior to your own, because you are imbalanced, and something is wrong with your body.

But what about the side effects of hormonal birth control? Did you know 63% of women go off the pill within the first year due to unwanted side effects? Not all women have bad experiences on the pill but the majority experience adverse side effects, sometimes without even realizing it for years until they stop and the "veil lifts."

ONE OTHER IMPORTANT ASPECT TO NOTE IS THAT THE PILL CAN ALTER YOUR NATURAL CHOICE IN A MATE.

It's true (primarily of heterosexual relationships): the pill can affect the type of man a woman is attracted to. The initial attraction to a male is all about pheromones and body odor. In a man's body scent lies hidden clues about his major histocompatibility complex (MHC) genes, which play an important role in immune system vigilance. Studies suggest that women prefer the scent of males whose MHC genes are genetically different or opposite of their own, a preference that most likely evolved to help offspring survive because couples with different MHC genes are less likely to be related. This means a lower chance of miscarriage, and their children are born with more varied MHC profiles and stronger immune systems. The problem is that the pill disrupts natural pheromones that guide you toward a genetically suitable mate. Studies have also shown men find women on the pill less attractive than those not on the pill due to copulins, which are cyclical pheromones specific to the vagina (when you are most fertile in the ovulatory phase) that draw sexual interest from men.

One study suggests that women on the pill undergo a shift in preference toward men who share similar MHC genes. Female subjects were more likely to rate the scent of a genetically similar man (via shirts worn by the men) as pleasant and

Common Side Effects of the Birth Control Pill

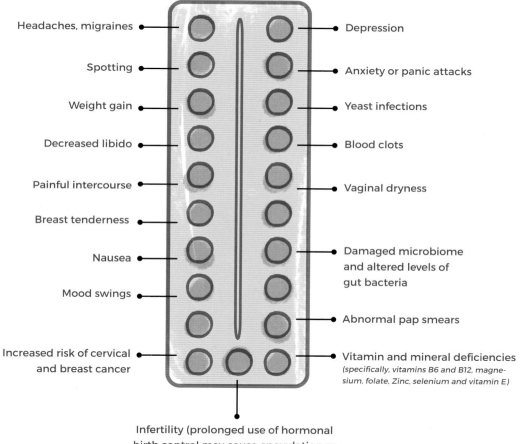

Headaches, migraines

Spotting

Weight gain

Decreased libido

Painful intercourse

Breast tenderness

Nausea

Mood swings

Increased risk of cervical and breast cancer

Depression

Anxiety or panic attacks

Yeast infections

Blood clots

Vaginal dryness

Damaged microbiome and altered levels of gut bacteria

Abnormal pap smears

Vitamin and mineral deficiencies
(specifically, vitamins B6 and B12, magnesium, folate, Zinc, selenium and vitamin E)

Infertility (prolonged use of hormonal birth control may cause anovulation or Amenorrhea, which can take months or years to regulate and which can cause temporary or permanent infertility)

desirable after they went on the pill, as compared to before. Scientists believe the hormonal changes that mimic pregnancy while on the pill draw women toward nurturing relatives, more so than a mate. Going off the pill while in a relationship may create some turmoil because you may not feel as sexually attracted to your partner as you once did while on the pill if he has a similar MHC-profile. You may even feel the urge to look elsewhere for a male with a MHC-profile different than yours. These findings are fascinating to me—that a tiny pill can influence sex, love, and marriage in more ways than one.

Your Period: The 5th Vital Sign

When you have a regular period, it serves as a monthly report card for what's happening in your body. For women, menstruation is our fifth vital sign. Here's what a natural period does for us:

- **PROVIDES HEALTH CLUES:** Without a natural period or cycle, you may miss the chance to address any imbalances or issues early on. Clues can be anything from the color of your period blood (see page 127), cramps, irregular periods, a cycle that is too short or too long, breast tenderness, painful periods, acne, mood swings, fatigue, weight gain, depression, high cholesterol, high blood pressure, and more. It's your body's way of telling you that it may not be balanced to its fullest extent. You will not experience these clues while on hormonal birth control.

- **NATURALLY CLEANSING:** Menstrual bleeding acts as a natural cleansing and waste removal process by releasing bacteria and discharging excess iron. Bleeding can also act as an emotional release and time to let go of anything or any thoughts that no longer serve you.

- **AWAKENS LIBIDO:** Oh, hello! Have we met before? During a natural cycle and leading up to ovulation, you will notice an increase in arousal and be naturally in the mood for sex (whether you want a baby or not). Not to mention, regular ovulation is associated with improved breast, bone, and heart health.

- **LONGEVITY:** Your natural period slows the aging process. Women age more slowly than men because of iron lost during menstruation, which also lowers your risk for cardiovascular disease, stroke, and Alzheimer's.

QUITTING THE PILL AND STARTING THE HAPPY HORMONE METHOD

There is no right or wrong way to come off the pill, but you have a couple of options. Keep in mind that everyone reacts differently. Unfortunately, stopping can bring back symptoms you had before you started the pill, along with new symptoms from your body trying to readjust without relying on synthetic hormones to do all the work. Your ovaries have been in hibernation and need to wake up.

Because of this, it's important to manage your expectations post-pill. Don't feel discouraged—the symptoms are temporary until your hormones sort themselves out with nutrition and lifestyle support. The adjustment period is inevitable and unavoidable so better to get it over with (at least in my opinion) because many rewards lie ahead.

I highly recommend starting the Happy Hormone Method 2–3 months before going off the pill. This will help you clean up your diet, reduce inflammation, heal your microbiome, eliminate endocrine-disrupting chemicals, and lay the foundation for your body to replenish lost micronutrient stores that you need to readjust and begin making your hormones again. Stopping the pill this way will help lessen the negative post-pill symptoms. You may not get your period back for a few months (it took mine six months to come back) but start by tracking any symptoms. You may experience PMS, temporary weight gain, hair loss, and post-pill acne (sometimes it's worse than before the pill), but in time and by sticking to this plan, symptoms should subside in a few months. Trust me; I've been there (except I didn't have a plan to guide me).

Think of the process as a chance to connect with your body, evaluate how it is reacting without the pill, notice how your real periods feel after having been asleep for so long, and open up the mind-body lines of communication. You can now see, feel and hear what's going on internally.

For a naturopathic method to help balance your cycle, facilitate the return of a period, and alleviate PMS symptoms, please refer to "Seed Cycling" on page 77.

Hormone-Based IUD's

A hormone-based IUD releases synthetic progestin in the uterus to thicken cervical mucus, preventing the survival of sperm and therefore, preventing pregnancy. While the amounts of synthetic hormones in these devices are far less than in oral contraceptives, ovulation and menstruation can still suppress, and the IUD interferes with natural hormone ratios. Any synthetic hormone you put in the body will come with side effects—it's as simple as that. A 2016 study revealed that the hormone-based IUD holds a higher risk of depression than the pill, which is something to consider.

NON-HORMONAL BIRTH CONTROL METHODS

The most important thing to remember as you consider this option is that you can only get pregnant 3-5 days of the month, during your fertile ovulation window.

Are you still sold on the fact that every time you have sex, you have a chance of getting pregnant? This false statement has been hammered into our brains since our first sex ed class and is entirely fear-based. The reality is, you can only get pregnant during your ovulation window when fertile mucus is present. Now, this gets complicated if you don't know your cycle, when you're ovulating, what type of cervical mucus to look for, or if you experience ovulation spotting (can be confused with a period but is unlikely), but it's easy to learn.

FERTILITY AWARENESS METHOD

This is what I use with the BBT method below. The Fertility Awareness Method is a natural, hormone-free method of birth control that involves learning to interpret fertile signs to know which days you are actually fertile. If you are trying to avoid pregnancy and you abstain from unprotected sex on the days you could possibly get pregnant, your chances of getting pregnant are slim to none. This is why, when the Fertility Awareness Method is used correctly, it is 99.4% effective. Start with the MyFLO tracker app (or your favorite tracking app; see page 221 for app recommendations) and begin to learn your cycle.

The MyFLO tracker app is pretty spot-on for me, as long as I'm checking in every day and entering my signs, symptoms, and periods. When you know you're ovulating (and don't want to get pregnant), practice safe sex and use a condom with spermicide, or avoid sex completely during the days before and after ovulation. Fertile mucus can keep sperm nourished and alive in your vagina for 3–5 days, so plan accordingly. There are plenty of fertile signs like cervical mucus, basal body temperature, and a few others that I talk about in the Ovulation chapter (page 175).

THE BBT METHOD (BASAL BODY TEMPERATURE)

The BBT method is most reliable when combined with the Fertility Awareness Method above. When used together, the two methods can have a success rate as high as 98 percent. This method is another way to pinpoint the day of ovulation so that you can avoid sex for the few days before and after peak ovulation days. It involves taking your basal body temperature (which means your temperature upon first waking every morning, before sitting up or doing anything) with an accurate "basal" thermometer (which is more precise than a regular thermometer). After ovulation takes place, a rise in temperature occurs for at least three consecutive days. You'll note this each month. This helps you figure out exactly when you're ovulating and recognize your fertility patterns.

You can use a basic digital basal thermometer (available online or at any drugstore), or a device like the Daysy which determines your fertile days and ovulation by recording, analyzing, and storing your temperature and menstrual cycle data over time. It will alert you on the days when intercourse may lead to pregnancy, including the day you ovulate and five days before ovulation.

Please see page 113 for a more detailed description of the BBT method.

MALE CONDOMS

Yes, condoms! When used correctly, condoms are 98% effective (just as effective as the pill) at preventing pregnancy. But people aren't perfect, and sometimes they aren't used correctly, which lowers their effective rate to 85%. For extra precaution, use condoms with spermicide, but only when you're ovulating.

COPPER IUD (NON-HORMONAL)

If you want an IUD, it's better to avoid the synthetic hormones and get the copper, hormone-free IUD. It releases a small amount of copper into the uterus to prevent sperm from fertilizing eggs. Sperm doesn't like copper, so this device makes it almost impossible for them to reach the egg.

This is an excellent option for many women because it doesn't suppress ovulation and you'll still experience real periods which means you can track each cycle phase, monitor your menstrual health, and reap the benefits of a natural cycle. It's over 99% effective for preventing pregnancy and lasts 12 years. There are some possible side effects to keep in mind. At the onset of use, it can cause heavy menstrual bleeding that usually subsides. Other possible side effects include heavier periods, cramping, pain during insertion, discomfort during sex, and spotting between periods.

FEMCAP

This is a reusable, latex-free cervical cap that is similar to a diaphragm but smaller. Shaped like a little sailor's cap, it fits around your cervix and can be left in for up to 48 hours for worry-free pregnancy prevention. The Femcap is over 92% effective and can be used in conjunction with a contraceptive gel (like ContraGel). Femcap comes in three different sizes. In the U.S., it must be fitted and prescribed by a doctor but is also available in some countries without a prescription.

CAYA DIAPHRAGM

Caya is a new one-size-fits-most reusable diaphragm that was designed to fit the female anatomy. It's made of silicone rather than latex and does not need to be fitted by your doctor. It's as safe as the original diaphragm but should always be used with a water-based contraceptive gel or spermicide such as ContraGel and should be left in after intercourse for at least 6 hours. It does require a prescription but can be filled by Caya directly through mail-order or at your local pharmacy.

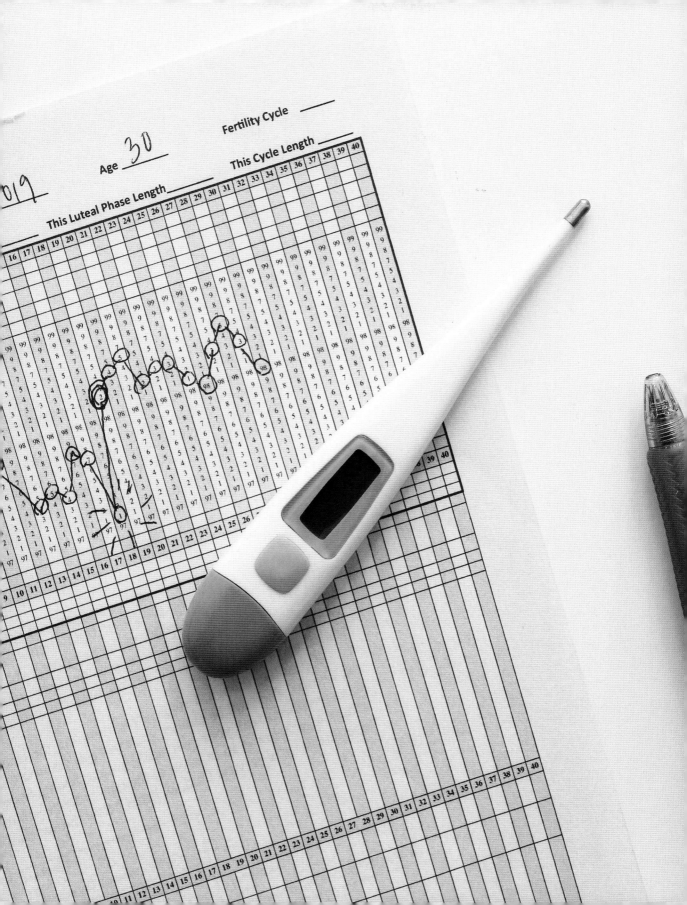

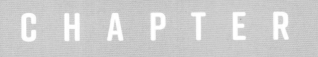

CHAPTER

4

PLANT-BASED NUTRITION

AS I'M SURE YOU'VE COME TO REALIZE, THERE are many layers and facets to your wellness journey. It is ever-changing as you learn, grow, and adapt. Food can act as healing medicine to naturally support and harmonize hormones, or it can act as a highly addictive and inflammatory drug. Either way, it's no secret that what you eat influences hormone function, how you look and feel, and your overall health.

The Happy Hormone Method celebrates feeding your body an abundance of fresh, high-vibrational, delicious, and seasonal plant foods containing nutrients that your cells can utilize. This means foods found in nature in their original, untouched form. They're unprocessed, free of chemicals and preservatives, and contain nothing artificial. These life-giving foods make up the infrastructure of a plant-based lifestyle and include an array of fresh vegetables, leafy greens, ripe fruits, gluten-free grains, legumes, nuts, and seeds. The colors you see in fresh produce represent vitamins unique to that fruit or vegetable, which is why eating a rainbow of plant foods ensures you are getting a variety of essential vitamins and minerals.

When you add in more of the right foods, there's less room in your diet for processed junk. Whole foods are full of fiber (essential for regular digestion/elimination, as mentioned earlier), water, vitamins, minerals, and enzymes, which allow us to feel satiated and full. Eating this way greatly reduces your risk for chronic diseases. Research suggests that eating a plant-based diet may reduce the risk for certain types of cancer and heart disease. It may help slow or prevent cognitive decline and Alzheimer's disease in older adults and can reduce the risk of developing diabetes while improving blood sugar control. Those who adopt a plant-based diet also tend to have smaller carbon footprints by helping reduce greenhouse gas emissions, land used for factory farming, and destruction of topsoil, while helping to conserve water and slow deforestation.

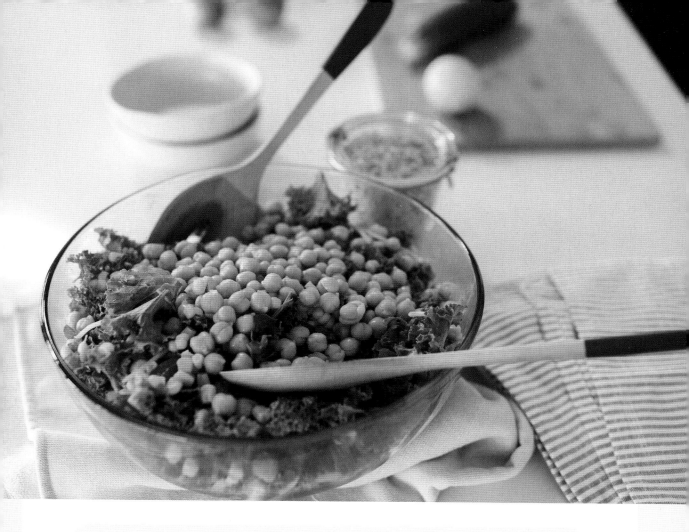

Environmental Impact—Some Facts:

- Eating one less burger each week is equivalent to taking your car off the road for 320 miles or line-drying your clothes half of the time.

- If a family of four skips meat and cheese one day each week, it's equivalent to your car off the road for five weeks or reducing everyone's daily showers by three minutes.

- If a family of four skips steak once a week, it's equivalent to taking your car off the road for nearly three months.

- If everyone in the U.S. removed meat or cheese from their diet just one day a week, it would be equivalent to driving 91 billion fewer miles or taking 7.6 million cars off the road.

Amazing changes are happening in the wellness realm, and a plant-based lifestyle is becoming more popular every day with grocery stores and restaurants offering products and menus that cater to plant-based diets. Doctors and health professionals have started writing "prescriptions" for more plants and fewer animal products because your cells thrive on alkalizing plant foods. A whole food, plant-based diet is also a powerful weight loss tool as it eliminates fast food, refined sugar, and refined grains.

EAT FOR YOUR CYCLE

We often get stuck in a routine when it comes to eating because it's convenient. We stick with what we know and like and end up eating the same foods week after week. Then we get bored or stressed out and throw in the towel. We order takeout more than we'd like or turn to processed meals because they're easy until we feel like being healthy again. And the cycle continues. Does that sound familiar? The problem with routine ways of eating is that your food can lack a variety of micronutrients necessary to fuel the functionality of your endocrine system and support hormone balance throughout each phase. You can even develop food sensitivities from regularly eating the same things.

Honestly, the food component of the Happy Hormone Method took months for me to grasp because I was very used to *my* way of eating. I remember feeling scared to branch out of my food bubble because I thought I was healthy, to begin with. Why do I have to change what I'm doing? How am I going to coordinate this every month? How am I going to remember what foods to eat and when? Then I thought about my debilitating PMS symptoms and terrible acne and fatigue and realized that whatever method I was following wasn't working for my hormones so trying something new was worth a shot. What did I have to lose?

Your body moves through four phases every single month, and the Happy Hormone Method will teach you how to eat (and live) in each phase to optimize your life and overall health.

Eating cyclically for your monthly cycle means switching up the types of foods you are consuming to optimize bodily functions at different times of the month. Eating this way ensures you consume a variety of necessary micronutrients and natural fiber from plants throughout the whole month. Every vegetable, fruit, legume, nut, and seed offers unique vitamins and minerals that can help your body flow through each phase with fewer symptoms and more energy to work on healing and restoration.

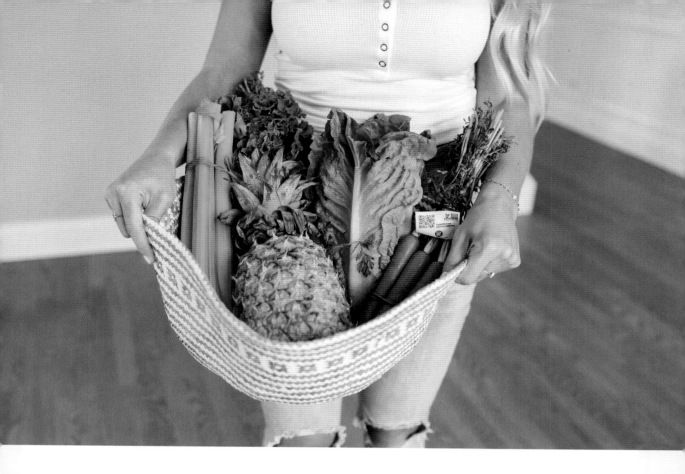

Once I fully committed to eating cyclically, I slowly created a new normal, and it made so much more sense than my prior eating habits. Sure, my old routine may have been "healthy," but it wasn't hormonally supportive. At first, it took some time to figure it all out. But this is precisely why I wrote *The Happy Hormone Guide*. I have it all mapped out for you in Part 2 of this book to make the transition as smooth and easy as possible.

This plan caters to women and aligns with what the body needs each week. Living this way keeps things exciting, ensures I'm eating a variety of foods, and prevents food boredom while also being comfortingly predictable.

IMPORTANCE OF BUYING ORGANIC PRODUCE—WHEN YOU CAN

Choosing organic produce is the best way to avoid endocrine-disrupting pesticides, toxic residue, GMO seed crops, and farming chemicals on your food. While eating a plant-based diet means you don't have to worry about hormones in meat or dairy products, it's important to consider the fruits and veggies you consume. I'm a huge believer in you get what you pay for, and if you aren't paying for it now, your health may pay for it later. While buying organic is more expensive, you are paying for the special care organic farmers place on protecting the environment. Organic farming practices prioritize health for the entire ecosystem, from healthy soil and crops, healthy animals, and a healthy environment for our planet.

Organic food is in its natural state, as it should be. Due to the strict standards, you know what you're getting because the food is traceable from farm to plate. Crops grown in organic soil have been shown to contain between 20 and 40 percent more antioxidants than conventional fruits and vegetables, but they do contain the same amounts of vitamins and minerals. Unlike conventional produce, organic produce grows with natural fertilizers and pesticides. Plus, organic crops aren't getting as much fertilizer as the more heavily sprayed conventional crops that grow at a faster rate. Organic farming practices vary but are backed by rigorous independent inspection and certifications.

With that said, I understand not everyone has the means to buy everything organic all the time. Fortunately, the EWG (Environmental Working Group) created recommendations for conscious shoppers called the *Dirty Dozen* and *Clean Fifteen*, with free guides you can download from their website and save to your phone or print out for reference. The *Dirty Dozen* lists the 12 most heavily sprayed fruits and veggies that you should always buy organic if you can. The *Clean Fifteen* lists fruits and veggies that you don't have to buy organic, for the current year. Each year, you'll want to refer to their website for updated lists. (https://www.ewg.org/)

How can you tell if a food is organic?

Look for the USDA Organic symbol on the tag or package, or you can check the barcode sticker on loose fruits and veggies. If the sticker contains five digits beginning with number nine, then it's organic. If there are only four digits, it's not organic.

HAPPY HORMONE MEALS

Happy Hormone meals do not lack in substance, color, or flavor. They align with the cycle phase you're in, offer a plentiful supply of macronutrients for satiety, and relatively small amounts of micronutrients for metabolism, hormone function, and overall wellness support.

Macronutrients are the protein, fats, and carbohydrates that make up your meals. Eating enough macronutrients convinces your hypothalamus that you are full and satiated, which turns off your hunger hormones (leptin and ghrelin) and prevents mindless grazing (which often stems from meals that aren't balanced or satisfying enough). This is important because your hypothalamus needs to feel that you are nourished enough to ovulate. It needs to know you are consuming enough calories and aren't in starvation mode (because that wouldn't be a good environment for a baby). As mentioned earlier, ovulation is the only way your body makes progesterone, and is essential for a healthy monthly cycle, even when you aren't trying to get pregnant (read more on why ovulation is important on page 177).

Micronutrients make up the essential vitamins, trace minerals, and phytonutrients of foods. Think of macronutrients as the foundation, walls, and roof of your house, and micronutrients as the kitchen, bathrooms, bedrooms, and closets that make up the inside, with all the things that make your house a home. Without macronutrients and micronutrients, your house would be incomplete.

This is how we begin to build balanced Happy Hormone meals. Before a meal, consider all of your nutritional bases. I make this easy in Part 2 by outlining the phase-specific foods to focus on with food charts and recommendations, as well as delicious recipes for breakfast, lunch, dinner, and dessert for each phase.

THE MACRONUTRIENT BREAKDOWN

Macronutrients contain the nutrition we need in larger amounts every day to thrive and have sustained energy throughout the day. The following sections on protein, fat, and complex carbohydrates explain why macros are important, how to incorporate them, and which foods represent the best sources for each. This is a basic overview until Part 2, when we dive into the specific sources to focus on how to optimize each cycle phase.

I. PROTEIN

Protein contains amino acids, which are the building blocks of life. You need protein for lean muscle health, bone health, hormone function, digestive enzymes,

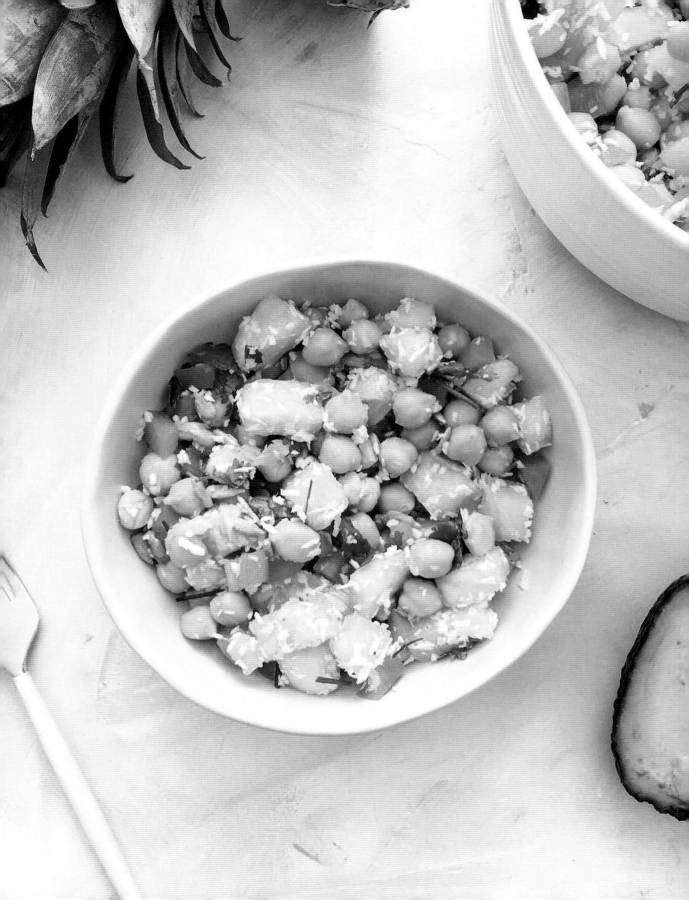

absorption of nutrients and repairing cells. Twenty amino acids are used to make protein in the body, and nine of them are essential amino acids we can only get from food (your body can synthesize the other 11). Every plant protein contains all nine essential amino acids, although some may be lower in certain amino acids than others. Contrary to what we used to believe, there is no need to combine proteins to make them more complete (like eating brown rice and black beans), because your body keeps an amino acid reserve, so it can fill in any gaps when necessary.

You can maximize your plant protein intake by eating a variety of legumes, whole grains, nuts and seeds, and some organic, minimally-processed soy. The protein recommendations for vegans are a little higher than the norm. A good estimate is to divide your body weight in half and aim to eat that number of grams of protein each day.

BEST PLANT PROTEIN SOURCES:

- ☐ Legumes: lentils, split peas, adzuki beans, black beans, navy beans, chickpeas, cannellini beans, northern beans, lima beans, mung beans, and kidney beans (minimally-processed options include chickpea pasta and lentil pasta)

- ☐ Vegetables: edamame, green peas, artichoke, nori sheets (seaweed)

- ☐ Nuts and seeds: almonds, brazil nuts, cashews, walnuts, hazelnuts, macadamia, pecans, peanuts, pumpkin seeds, sunflower seeds, flaxseed, chia seeds, sesame seeds, hemp seeds

- ☐ Whole grains: quinoa, amaranth, brown rice, buckwheat, gluten-free oats

- ☐ Organic soy products (in moderation): tofu, tempeh, natto

- ☐ Protein powders: make sure all ingredients are sourced from whole foods only, with minimal or no added sugar, zero artificial sweeteners, and zero fillers. My favorite vegan brands are Vega, 22 Days Nutrition, Garden of Life, Nutiva, Sprout Living, and Owyn.

2. FAT

Fats are essential for brain function, hormone production, metabolism, energy, immunity, and inflammatory response. Your hormones love healthy fats. They are necessary for proper nutrient absorption and even keep us feeling satiated after meals.

There are two types of fats: saturated and unsaturated. Saturated fats are found mainly in animal sources, except for coconut and coconut oil. Unsaturated fats are mostly found in plants. Within unsaturated fats, there are monounsaturated fatty acids and polyunsaturated fatty acids, both of which are thought to lower bad LDL cholesterol. It's important to keep in mind that real, whole foods contain a mix of fatty acids, so we can't get too hung up on the differences. For example, avocado is made up of mainly monounsaturated fatty acids, a small amount of polyunsaturated fatty acids, and an even smaller amount of saturated fat.

Within the polyunsaturated fatty acids are a group called omega-3 and omega-6 fatty acids, and both are essential to your health (except that Americans often way over-consume omega-6 fatty acids as they are rampant in processed foods and processed vegetable oils). Omegas from real foods can lower inflammation, reduce triglycerides and plaque in the blood, and nourish the brain by preventing memory loss and depression. Broken down even further, there are two forms of omega-3's that are most beneficial; these are DHA and EPA, mostly found in fatty fish. For plant-based eaters, there are sources of omegas that your body can further break down into DHA and EPA found in flaxseed, chia seeds, hemp seeds, edamame, walnuts, and beans. You may want to consider supplementing DHA and EPA from a vegan, algae-derived supplement (like Algae Omega from Nordic Naturals).

As you will see, the Happy Hormone Method incorporates fats into each phase. We don't skimp on fats. They are especially high in the follicular phase (avocados are one of the top ovulation-supporting foods), but we love on them throughout each phase. That said, it's easy to overdo it on nuts, seeds, and almond butter, because they're so darn delicious. So yes, they are healthy but keep them to reasonable portions (approximately a third cup per day).

BEST FAT SOURCES:

- ☐ Avocados

- ☐ Olives

- ☐ Coconut

- ☐ Nuts and seeds (almonds, brazil nuts, cashews, walnuts, hazelnuts, macadamia, pecans, peanuts, pumpkin seeds, sunflower seeds, flaxseed, chia seeds, sesame seeds, hemp seeds)

- ☐ Raw nut and seed butter (almond butter, cashew butter, peanut butter, sunflower seed butter, coconut butter, and tahini)

- ☐ Oils (avocado, coconut, grapeseed, olive)

3. COMPLEX CARBOHYDRATES AND FIBER

This is a difficult subject because people are either scared of carbs, overdo them, eat the wrong kinds, or have a healthy relationship with them. I don't know where you stand. What I will say is that a low-carb or keto diet does not work for every-one. I recommend quitting sugar and wheat before carbs, as you'll see below.

With the Happy Hormone Method, we add complex carbohydrate sources, more in the luteal and menstrual phases when the body needs them, and then in moder-ate amounts in the follicular and ovulatory phases when you already have increased energy and don't necessarily need as much energy from carb sources. A long term, low-carb diet can lead to anovulatory cycles or hypothalamic amenorrhea, espe-cially if your HPA axis is out of whack from high stress. Certain carbohydrate sources have a calming effect on your nervous system, which is essential for heal-ing from HPA Axis Dysregulation and can improve the cortisol response in highly stressed people.

The complex carbs come from beans and legumes, whole grains (like quinoa and rice) and starchy vegetables. They have adequate fiber, are unrefined, and do not contain gluten (because it's highly inflammatory). So that I don't lose my sanity, I have sourdough bread made locally (the real kind with yeast in the ingre-dients instead of a sourdough starter). While it does contain gluten, it also has the added digestive benefits from fermentation and was not made in a factory. I'll also have a gluten-free pasta made from rice, kelp, chickpeas, edamame or lentils and occasionally almond flour crackers or rice cakes. Other than that, my meals center around whole, unprocessed foods.

BEST COMPLEX CARBOHYDRATE SOURCES:

- **WHOLE GRAINS:** quinoa, brown rice, jasmine rice, basmati rice, black rice, wild rice, millet, buckwheat, gluten-free oats (yes, they exist)

- **STARCHY VEGETABLES:** sweet potatoes, butternut squash, acorn squash, corn, yams, pumpkin

- **LEGUMES:** lentils, split peas, adzuki beans, black beans, navy beans, chickpeas, cannellini beans, northern beans, lima beans, mung beans, and kidney beans (minimally processed options include chickpea pasta and lentil pasta)

HIGH FIBER HAPPY HORMONE FOODS:

Navy beans, lentils, pinto beans, tempeh, artichokes, green peas, green leafy veg-etables, chia seeds, flax seeds, raspberries, avocado, chickpeas, lima beans, black beans, broccoli, pears, apples, figs, pumpkin seeds, pistachios, almonds, prunes, edamame, and sweet potatoes

THE MICRONUTRIENT BREAKDOWN

While you need much smaller amounts of micronutrients than you do macronutrients, they are equally important for hormone function. The following are lists sourced from the USDA and veganhealth.org, with the best food sources for each vitamin and mineral, and the recommended daily amounts for women. *Note: daily amounts will vary if you are pregnant or breastfeeding.* This is a basic overview until Part 2 when we dive into the specific vitamins and minerals for each phase and those that vegans/plant-based eaters need to be aware of to prevent a deficiency.

ESSENTIAL VITAMINS

☐ **VITAMIN A (BETA CAROTENE)** 700 mcg daily: sweet potatoes, carrots, pumpkins, squash, spinach, mangos, turnip greens

☐ **VITAMIN B1 (THIAMINE)** 1.5 mg daily: brown rice, soymilk, watermelon, acorn squash, hibiscus tea, sunflower seeds, tahini, macadamia nuts, spirulina, nutritional yeast, bakers yeast, soybeans

☐ **VITAMIN B2 (RIBOFLAVIN)** 1.7 mg daily: green leafy vegetables, quinoa, buckwheat, almonds, spinach, mushrooms, beet greens

☐ **VITAMIN B3 (NIACIN)** 20 mg daily: coffee, nutritional yeast, peanuts, peanut butter, mushrooms, potatoes, spirulina, chili powder, barley, tomatoes, chia seeds, wild rice, buckwheat, avocados, green peas

☐ **VITAMIN B5 (PANTOTHENIC ACID)** 10 mg daily: mushrooms, avocado, tomatoes, paprika, sunflower seeds, broccoli, sweet potatoes, nutritional yeast

☐ **VITAMIN B6 (PYRIDOXINE)** 2 mg daily: organic tofu and soy products, bananas, legumes, squash, pumpkin, watermelon, almonds, sweet potatoes with skin, hemp seeds, prunes, pineapple, chickpeas, artichoke hearts, water chestnuts, figs, kale, collards

☐ **VITAMIN B7 (BIOTIN)** 300 mcg daily: avocados, almonds, walnuts, peanuts, chia seeds, sweet potatoes, onions, oats, tomatoes, carrots

☐ **VITAMIN B9 (FOLATE/FOLIC ACID)** 400 mcg daily: organic soybeans, whole grains, beans, lentils, asparagus, avocados, celery, cauliflower, mangos, oranges, cantaloupe, walnuts, flax, sesame, tahini, mint

☐ **VITAMIN B12 (METHYLCOBALAMIN)** 1500 mcg daily: spirulina, nutritional yeast, fortified soy products, fortified almond milk

☐ **VITAMIN C (ASCORBIC ACID)** 75 mg daily: citrus, bell peppers, broccoli, potatoes, strawberries, spinach, Brussels sprouts, tomatoes

☐ **VITAMIN D (CHOLECALCIFEROL)** 2,000 IU daily: mushrooms, fortified soy and almond milk, tofu, sunlight(!)

☐ **VITAMIN E (TOCOPHEROLS)** 15 mg daily: cucumber, vegetable oils, leafy greens, whole grains, almonds, hazelnuts, sunflower seeds, wheat germ

☐ **VITAMIN K (PHYLLOQUINONE)** 90 mcg daily: cabbage, spinach, broccoli, sprouts, kale, collards

ESSENTIAL MINERALS

☐ **CALCIUM** 1000 mcg daily: tofu, collards, mustard greens, turnip greens, kale, bok choy, tempeh, broccoli, Swiss chard, sesame seeds, tahini, fortified nut milk, dried figs, edamame, navy beans, pinto beans, oats

☐ **CHLORIDE** 2.3 g daily: sea salt, seaweed (kelp), olives, rye, tomatoes, lettuce, celery

☐ **CHROMIUM** 120 mcg daily: broccoli, potatoes, oats, kale, spirulina

☐ **COPPER** 2 mg daily: sesame seeds, cashews, edamame, mushrooms, beet greens, turnip greens, spinach, asparagus, cacao, prunes, black pepper, sunflower seeds, tempeh, chickpeas, lentils, walnuts, lima beans

☐ **FLUORIDE** 3 mg daily: black tea, oolong, white, green tea, kombucha

☐ **IODINE** 150 mcg daily; seaweed (kelp), iodized salt, Marine Coast Kelp Granules Sea Seasoning (can be found at Whole Foods), prunes

☐ **IRON** 18 mg daily: cooked spinach, cooked Swiss chard, tofu, tempeh, lentils, kidney beans, black beans, edamame, black-eyed peas, beets and beet greens, quinoa, potato, tahini, green peas, blackstrap molasses, cashews

☐ **MAGNESIUM** 400 mg daily: dark chocolate, avocados, hemp seeds, cashews, sunflower seeds, tofu, legumes, quinoa, almonds, summer squash, kelp, oats

☐ **MANGANESE** 2 mg daily: oats, brown rice, chickpeas, cloves, cinnamon, pineapple, spinach, collard greens, raspberries, strawberries, turmeric, garlic, basil, bok choy

☐ **MOLYBDENUM** 75 mcg daily: green peas, lentils, black beans, kidney beans, lima beans, pinto beans, oats, cucumber, celery, tomatoes

☐ **PHOSPHORUS** 1,000 mg daily: soybeans, pumpkin seeds, lentils, tempeh, mushrooms, tofu, green peas, broccoli, asparagus, Brussels sprouts, cauliflower, fennel, summer squash, Swiss chard

☐ **POTASSIUM** 3,500 mg daily: bok choy, Swiss chard, beet greens, Brussels sprouts, tomatoes, cabbage, spinach, sweet potatoes, mushrooms, celery, papaya, cantaloupe, banana, carrots, oranges, kale

☐ **SELENIUM** 70 mcg daily: brazil nuts, mushrooms, asparagus, mustard seeds, tofu, brown rice, sunflower seeds, sesame seeds

☐ **SODIUM** 1,500-2,300 mg daily: sea salt, pickles, soy sauce, tamari, beets, Swiss chard, celery, sweet potatoes

☐ **SULFUR** daily amount unknown: broccoli, cabbage, cauliflower, Brussels sprouts, kale, leeks, bok choy, garlic, onion, shallots, chives

☐ **ZINC** 25 mg daily: sesame seeds, asparagus, mushrooms, pumpkin seeds, chickpeas, lentils, cashews, quinoa

Minimally-Processed Soy Products

Soy products that are minimally processed include edamame, tempeh, tofu, natto, miso, and tamari (not processed, textured, soy protein, fake meat products or soy protein isolate).

Soy products have high levels of phytoestrogens. If you have estrogen-dominant conditions (like PCOS, endometriosis or fibroids) you want to avoid soy products in the ovulatory and luteal phases (outlined in Part 2) and avoid or limit soy products to smaller amounts in the menstrual and follicular phases. This is because you have trouble breaking down estrogen as is, so adding phytoestrogens (which act like natural estrogen) could make matters even worse. On the contrary, if you are in menopause, then phytoestrogens are highly beneficial for you so no need to worry about limiting amounts.

If you are not in menopause, small amounts of minimally-processed soy can be beneficial for health in general. So, they are great to eat during your menstrual and follicular phases (in moderate amounts) if you want to reap the health benefits. Plus, they are great sources of plant protein.

Steer clear of soy milk, soy yogurts, soy cheeses, and processed, vegan meats. As most soy products are likely to be GMO, it's important to buy them organic.

HOME COOKING

Unless you already cook most of your food, the thought of cooking more may feel new and intimidating, but we all have to start somewhere. The truth is that cooking your own food is fundamental for any health journey. Otherwise, you end up relying on others who may not have your best interest at heart and may add in unnecessary or harmful ingredients you are unaware of like vegetable oils, excessive sodium or sugar, and processed ingredients.

You most definitely do not have to be a trained chef to make my recipes or follow this plan. I'm a self-taught home cook. All you need are basic cooking skills like chopping, steaming, boiling, and sautéing. Sure, cooking your own food is more time-consuming but that's the reality of any healthy lifestyle, and creating new habits around cooking is the key to success. We're all short on time, so I aim to keep Happy Hormone meals simple and easy enough for anyone to follow.

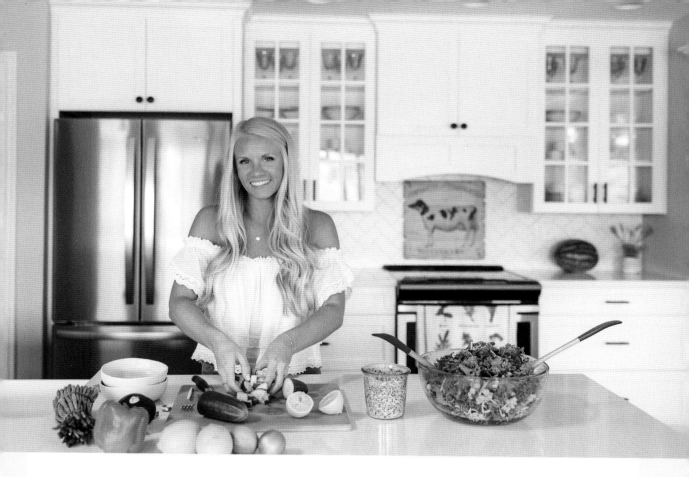

KEEP YOUR PANTRY AND FREEZER STOCKED

Having a well-stocked pantry and freezer allows for quick and easy meals. In the pantry, I love to stay stocked up on assorted beans, lentils, brown rice, quinoa, crushed tomatoes, veggie broth, canned coconut milk, dried herbs and spices, nutritional yeast, nuts and seeds, vegan protein powder, almond flour, dates, and vegan chocolate chips. In the freezer, I make sure to have shelled edamame, ready-to-steam jasmine rice, riced cauliflower, riced broccoli, riced carrots, mixed veggies for stir fry, fruit for smoothies, and sprouted or gluten-free bread.

COOKING OILS

Every oil has a smoke point, which is the maximum temperature it can be heated while cooking before it starts to smoke. If oil begins smoking, the nutritious minerals in the oil have broken down and began to oxidize, creating carcinogens and free radicals that are toxic when consumed. At this point, the oil will also produce a chemical called acrolein which makes burnt food taste bitter and smell unpleasant.

An oil's smoke point temperature is highly affected by its fatty acid profile, meaning its ratio of saturated fat to monounsaturated and polyunsaturated fat, and how refined it is.

Avoid refined and processed vegetable oils like:

- ☐ Canola oil
- ☐ Corn oil
- ☐ Soybean oil
- ☐ Sunflower oil
- ☐ Cottonseed oil
- ☐ Sesame oil
- ☐ Safflower oil

Cook and bake with high-heat oils like:

- ☐ Coconut oil (for baking)
- ☐ Avocado oil (for frying and grilling)
- ☐ Grapeseed, avocado or coconut oil (for lightly sautèing)

For dipping and sauce, use a low-temperature oil that has a great flavor like:

- ☐ Extra-virgin olive oil
- ☐ Flaxseed oil
- ☐ Walnut oil

SOAKING NUTS AND SEEDS

Nuts and seeds add a variety of fiber, protein, vitamins, and minerals to a plant-based diet, but sometimes eating them raw can be hard on your digestion. By soaking your raw nuts and seeds before eating, you can enhance their nutritional profile and digestibility. Soak them in a bowl or mason jar with filtered water for 7-8 hours. This activates and releases their enzyme inhibitors and phytates, which makes them easier to absorb and digest. Be sure to drain, rinse, and then dry them completely afterward, so they don't turn moldy. You'll notice how they plump up after being soaked. Soak, drain, rinse, dry, and eat. You can also store them in the refrigerator to maintain freshness and prevent them from going rancid.

SEED CYCLING

Seed cycling refers to a naturopathic method of rotating different seeds throughout different times of your menstrual cycle. Doing this can support hormone balance which, in turn, may alleviate those pesky PMS symptoms like acne, amenorrhea, heavy bleeding, fatigue, infertility, insomnia, and others. Different seeds provide various oils, vitamins, and minerals that can help stimulate production, detox-ification, and metabolism of estrogen and progesterone. The alternating seeds include flax, pumpkin, sesame, and sunflower seeds.

- ☐ Ground flaxseeds are more easily absorbed than whole flaxseeds, so you should always grind them (otherwise you'll poop them out whole).
  Note: If you are grinding flax seeds, do not soak them first because they'll turn into a wet mess.

- ☐ Pumpkin, sesame, or sunflower seeds can be eaten raw, raw and soaked, or raw and ground.

- ☐ Nuts and seeds can go rancid if not stored properly, so it's best to refrigerate them in glass jars to keep them fresh.

DAY 1–13
ESTROGEN BOOST

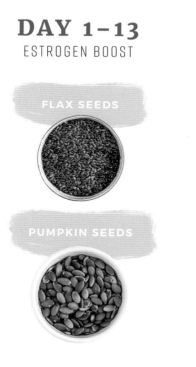

FLAX SEEDS

PUMPKIN SEEDS

DAY 14–28
PROGESTERONE BOOST

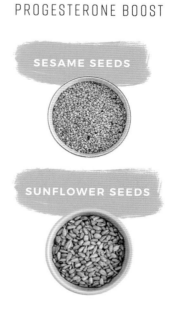

SESAME SEEDS

SUNFLOWER SEEDS

HOW TO SEED CYCLE

In Part 2, each phase incorporates seed cycling, so no need to memorize the following information, but I wanted to provide a basic overview of how and why it works. I've been following the seed cycling method for a while and think it's a wonderful place to start eating for your cycle because it's effective and easy to incorporate.

Seed cycling divides into two rotations. Even if your cycle is irregular and does not fall within the average 28 to 30-day range, I recommend working off of the days in a normal menstrual cycle because this will gently encourage your cycle to balance itself out.

The first rotation combines your menstrual and follicular phases (days 1–14), to support rising estrogen levels with flaxseeds and pumpkin seeds. Here's how they work:

- Flax seeds are high in phytoestrogens that promote estrogen production as well as lignans that help detoxify excess estrogens and fiber to eliminate them. Together, they work to harmonize optimal estrogen ratios.

- Flax seeds and pumpkin seeds are rich in omega-3 fatty acids that fight inflammation and work to regulate FSH levels for ovulation support, not to mention their amazing benefits for healthy skin, hair, and nails.

- Pumpkin seeds (or pepitas) are high in zinc, which helps prime and support the production of adequate progesterone in the next phase (the luteal phase).

Add flaxseeds to smoothies, chia pudding, energy balls, oatmeal or baked goods. Add pumpkin seeds to salads, yogurt bowls, or homemade trail mix.

The second rotation combines your ovulatory and luteal phases (days 15–28) to support progesterone levels with sesame seeds and sunflower seeds. Here's how they work:

- Sesame seeds are high in lignans, which help harmonize and modulate estrogen levels. They're also rich in magnesium and calcium to ease PMS cramps and provide an immunity boost.

- Both sesame seeds and sunflower seeds are high in omega-6 fatty acids, which help reduce PMS-related inflammation while also supporting progesterone levels.

- Sunflower seeds are rich in selenium, which is essential for liver function, to ensure proper detoxification and elimination of excess hormones and magnesium.

Add sesame and sunflower seeds to salads, soups, stir-fries, sauces, baked goods, or energy balls.

Seed cycling is a simple, natural, and inexpensive way to support fluctuating hormones.

See my Seed Cycling Snack Balls recipe on page 218.

Finding Your Happy Weight

This isn't a weight loss book, but weight may be correlated with hormone balance. Sometimes, gaining a little weight may be beneficial for your body to achieve healthy hormone function. The same goes for losing weight. As women, we have to find, accept and embrace our happy weight, whatever it may be, instead of going against where our body wants to be. Our culture is changing and what matters more than the number on the scale is our health and our natural shape. Otherwise, we are constantly swimming upstream and getting nowhere in terms of our physical, mental, or emotional health.

The Happy Hormone Guide will help you find your happy weight, whether your body wants to gain or lose, to find its sweet spot. Through intuitive eating, following hunger cues, giving your body nourishment it wants and needs throughout the month and doing the corresponding workouts, your weight will work itself out over time. The numbers should not be a focal point when it comes to balancing hormones. When you honor your body with the lifestyle action steps in chapter 6 and follow the Happy Hormone Method throughout your cycle, things will fall into place naturally.

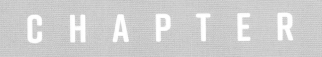

CHAPTER

5

SUPPLEMENTS & HEALING HERBS

N A PERFECT WORLD, WE COULD GET EVERYTHING WE NEED from food alone. But nowadays, the soil that grows our food is often depleted of nutrients due to modern farming practices. I'm not going to pretend that every vegan is healthy and gets what they need from food alone. Because there is not much we can do about our food system in the U.S. (except to buy more organic produce), we should focus on getting the nutrients we need to be able to maintain our vegan or plant-based lifestyles. Some people have a harder time absorbing nutrients, and supplementation can help fill in the gaps. Supplementing also becomes highly beneficial in times of stress, when vitamins and minerals quickly deplete.

Supplementation and healing herbs will only work alongside a nourishing, plant-forward diet and healthy lifestyle that includes exercise, high-quality sleep, and healthy stress management.

The supplements and herbs you decide to take will *not* outwork a poor diet, excessive alcohol consumption, lack of sleep, overuse of endocrine-disrupting products, or poor gut health. You can't take one supplement in the hopes that it will balance your hormones without changing anything else.

Before starting a new supplement or herb protocol, I urge you to get hormone and nutrient level testing done (refer to the Hormone Testing section on page 32), so you are not guessing or wasting money on herbs or supplements. Always talk to your doctor or naturopath before starting new supplementation.

THE PLANT-BASED ESSENTIALS

As much as people don't want to hear it, there are certain vitamins and minerals to be aware of when you stop eating animal foods to avoid the risk of deficiencies. Even if you eat a clean, healthy, whole food diet, it's unlikely that you are consuming enough of every vitamin and mineral from food alone (this can be true for meat eaters, as well). The Happy Hormone Method encourages variety, which will help increase your intake of these vital nutrients from food sources as well as supplementation to fill in the gaps.

An excellent way to measure your current nutrient intake from food is to enter everything you eat every day for a week, into an app like Cronometer that calculates whether or not you are meeting the daily requirements. This will give you a good idea of where you may be lacking and can act as a starting point for creating a supplement protocol (in addition to working with your doctor or naturopath). It is recommended to try a new protocol for three months before stopping or giving up, because it takes 100 days for new follicles to develop, and for you to begin noticing improvements. Also, wait three months before incorporating new herb or supplement protocols.

Each time you get your hormone and nutrient levels tested is a great time to reassess your supplement protocol and make adjustments as necessary.

Figuring out the supplements to incorporate will depend on your genetics, current hormone and nutrient levels, the variety of foods in your diet, how well you absorb nutrients, current stress levels, and gut health. I do not know where you stand, but the following includes essential vitamins and minerals that are crucial for hormone balance in women (ages 18–65) and is sourced from the USDA and veganhealth.org. These will support estrogen and progesterone production and can significantly improve your period and hormone health while reducing PMS symptoms and promoting overall health.

Note: Multi-vitamins usually contain more of what we don't need and less of what we do need. For instance, I highly doubt your multi-vitamin has magnesium glycinate, iodine, and selenium, let alone in the right amounts—all of which are essential for hormone balance. I prefer to get most of the nutrients that are in multi-vitamins (like vitamins A and C and calcium) from food sources, and then supplement with the following essentials separately, or as needed.

B VITAMINS

B vitamins are essential to help the liver eliminate excess estrogen each month, which will help reduce PMS symptoms. Vitamin B6 in particular, helps synthesize progesterone, makes red blood cells, reduces inflammation, reduces bloat, and reduces overproduction of sebum (which will help those with acne and oily skin). Vitamin B12 is a non-negotiable for vegans because the amount of B12 found in plant-based foods is not enough to meet your body's needs. Because our livers become depleted of B vitamins so quickly, it's important to adequately replenish our supply since they provide the energy our cells need for fuel. I prefer a B-complex that contains all of the activated B vitamins, like the Country Life Coenzyme B-Complex Caps or B-Right from Jarrow Formulas. I also love the highly absorbable VeganSafe B-12 Bioactive drops for extra energy, especially in my luteal phase.

Here are the daily recommendations (sourced from the USDA and veganhealth. org) for each B vitamin (for some, the amounts will be higher in a supplement form, for higher absorption rates):

VITAMIN B1 (THIAMINE)	1.5 mg
VITAMIN B2 (RIBOFLAVIN)	1.7 mg
VITAMIN B3 (NIACIN)	20 mg
VITAMIN B5 (PANTOTHENIC ACID)	10 mg
VITAMIN B6 (PYRIDOXINE)	2 mg
VITAMIN B7 (BIOTIN)	300 mcg
VITAMIN B9 (FOLATE)	400 mcg
VITAMIN B12 (METHYLCOBALAMIN)	1500 mcg

Note: If you think vitamin B12 makes your skin break out, it could be the methylcobalamin form. Try the cyanocobalamin form which is the synthetic version but is less likely to make you break out (2.4 mcg daily).

MAGNESIUM CHELATE (MAGNESIUM GLYCINATE)

Magnesium is an essential mineral needed for 300+ chemical reactions in the body, and most women (and men) are deficient because day-to-day stress uses up magnesium stores like crazy. It's a front-line treatment for almost every period symptom and hormonal problem under the sun including PMS, PCOS, thyroid conditions, perimenopause, HPA Axis Dysregulation, anxiety, insomnia, and high

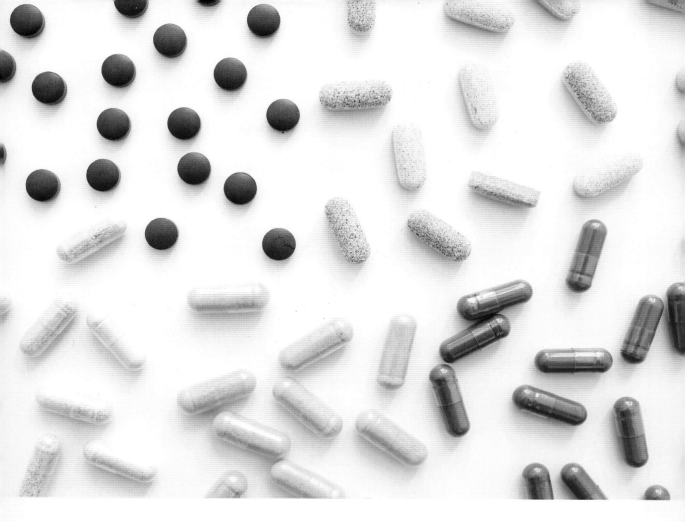

cortisol. Magnesium works together with vitamin B6 to manufacture progesterone. It reduces inflammation and calms the nervous system which is why you almost instantly feel relaxed and calm after taking it.

Food sources of magnesium are usually not enough to meet daily levels because we deplete them so quickly. Magnesium chelate (or magnesium glycinate) is the best and most absorbable form to restore magnesium levels. Magnesium Citrate (which is what the CALM magnesium tea is formulated from), is more for digestion-related issues like constipation or bloating and can cause an upset stomach, so keep that in mind. Also, there is no way to test magnesium levels, but the general recommendation is that if you are a human living in today's busy world, you need more magnesium. I take Magnesium Glycinate before bed because it puts me right to sleep. The recommended daily amount is 400 mg. I like Solgar Chelated Magnesium or Viva Naturals Magnesium Biglycinate.

VITAMIN D

You can obtain vitamin D through non-dairy milk and direct sunlight exposure (without sunscreen) to enhance your body's natural vitamin D production, but if you live in a cold climate or have fair skin, it can be difficult to source enough of this nutrient through food alone. Vegans can have an especially hard time, which is why I highly recommend supplementing vitamin D. If you have inflammation or a magnesium deficiency, vitamin D production is inhibited which is problematic because both are essential for hormone function. You also need vitamin D for calcium absorption and healthy bones. Be sure to look for a supplement that's labeled vegan, as many D3 supplements are animal-derived. The recommended daily amount is 2,000 IU. I like the Suntrex D3 drops from Global Healing Center or Country Life Vegan D3 supplements.

ZINC

Zinc is an essential mineral that our bodies cannot store, so it's important to eat foods high in zinc or take a zinc supplement. Zinc is crucial for estrogen production and healthy maturation of follicles. Healthy follicles promote ovulation. Ovulation helps make progesterone in your luteal phase, and adequate levels of progesterone help regulate your cycle overall while reducing PMS symptoms. Zinc is wonderful for your skin because it's anti-inflammatory, helps maintain collagen and healthy connective tissue, and clears up acne, not to mention its immunity-boosting effects. When I start to feel sick, I will double my daily dose of zinc to boost immune function. I like the Solgar Zinc Citrate or Garden of Life Vitamin Code Raw Zinc. The recommended daily amount is 25 mg of zinc citrate.

IODINE AND SELENIUM

Iodine is an essential mineral that's crucial for thyroid hormone production, immunity, and brain function. It also plays a significant role in breast and ovary health, as it protects you from estrogen overload by down-regulating estrogen receptors. Iodine has been shown to significantly reduce fibrocystic breast changes and decrease the risk of breast cancer. Iodine is also a treatment for breast tenderness, breast cysts, ovarian cysts, heavy periods, fluid retention, and ovulation pain. It's important to pair iodine with selenium, as it protects your thyroid from over-stimulation and damage.

Note: If you have a thyroid condition, do your research and speak to your doctor about iodine supplementation.

I recommend liquid iodine in the form of potassium iodide drops or Nascent Iodine drops. I like the Detoxadine drops from Global Healing Center or the drops from Benevolent Nourishment (or any potassium iodide drops from your local health food store). The daily recommended amount is 150 mcg.

Pair it with selenium, which is also an essential mineral, in the form of 1–2 raw brazil nuts per day (one brazil nut contains roughly 90 mcg of selenium). The daily recommended amount of selenium is 70 mcg.

Note: You can also get iodine through sprinkling kelp granules (I like the Sea Seasoning brand) on your food.

IRON

Iron is an essential mineral. We need iron to make healthy oxygen-carrying red blood cells, transport oxygen from the lungs to organs and tissues throughout the body, to support thyroid hormones and for reproduction. I try to consume as much iron as possible from food sources, but I still take an iron supplement for overall health and well-being, especially since I'm vegan. If you feel fatigued or have difficulty focusing, shortness of breath, pale skin, difficulty staying warm, lack of endurance, muscle weakness, prolonged soreness, heart palpitations, brittle or ridged nails, or if you get sick often, you may be low in iron. Talk to your doctor if you think you may have an iron deficiency because it's important to get your levels checked.

I like the Megafood Blood Builder supplement or the Garden of Life Vitamin Code Raw Iron. The daily recommended amount of iron is 18 mg for women ages 18–65.

PROBIOTIC

A daily probiotic is beneficial for rebalancing your gut flora, keeping the bacteria happy, and reducing inflammation. This will help reduce bloating and promote daily bowel movements, which eliminate excess estrogen. There are hundreds of probiotic brands out there, but my favorites are the Renew Life (the Extra Care 50 billion is vegan) or the Up4 Ultra Probiotics. There is no daily recommended amount for probiotics, but anywhere from 20–50 billion cultures with at least 12 strains is sufficient.

OMEGA-3 ALGAE-DERIVED DHA/EPA

Many dietitians recommend supplementing a vegan diet with DHA or EPA because omega-3 fatty acids are harder to source through plant-based foods than animal proteins. DHA and EPA play an important role in fighting inflammation while also supporting mood, brain health, and heart health. I prefer to get my omega-3's through flax seeds, chia seeds, and walnuts, but also supplement with the Nested Naturals Vegan Omega-3 or the DEVA Omega-3 DHA supplement. The recommended amount is 250 mg daily of algae-derived long-chain omega-3's (EPA/DHA).

What Are Adaptogens?

Adaptogens come in many forms, from pills and extracts to powders and blends. Adaptogens are amazing plants that tend to grow in the most inhospitable areas of the earth: deserts, cold mountains, dry and barren land. Some even date back to the ice age. Living in such harsh conditions, adaptogenic plants have developed a surreal resiliency to survive environmental stressors. When we consume these adaptogens, our body's ability to deal with stress in our internal and external environments greatly improves. Adaptogens do not serve one single function; instead, they adapt to whatever your body needs help with at the time and work to alleviate the symptoms. Most of the adaptogens I'm sharing with you are pretty standard. I've found that they greatly help my ability to deal with stress. I include different adaptogens in the symptom-specific supplement and herb section, but feel free to do your own research and incorporate more based on your body's unique needs.

SYMPTOM-SPECIFIC HERBS & SUPPLEMENTS

The plant-based essentials in the last section are the most important forms of supplementation for happy hormones and should be incorporated before adding any of the following, which are bonuses that can promote holistic healing and alleviate unwanted symptoms. Multiple options are included for each symptom, but this doesn't mean you should take them all at the same time. Talk to your doctor first, do your research and then choose the additional herbs and supplements that could work best for you.

SEVERE PMS

- Vitex Chaste Tree Berry (not suitable for all types of PCOS)
- Rhodiola
- DIM (diindolylmethane), like Estroblock Pro
- Dong Quai
- Shatavari

AMENORRHEA AND OVULATION SUPPORT

- Vitex (Chaste-Tree Berry)
- Evening Primrose Oil
- Ashwagandha
- Maca powder (the red variety)
- Inositol

PERIOD CRAMPS

- Cramp Bark
- Reishi
- CBD Oil (from high-quality brands such as Charlotte's web or NuLeaf Naturals)
- Saje Wellness Moon Cycle Soothing Oil Blend (apply to the lower abdomen and lower back)

THYROID SUPPORT

- Magic Moss by SOL Solutions (contains sea moss, bladderwrack, dandelion)
- Ashwagandha
- L-tyrosine
- Sea vegetables (nori, kelp, dulse)

LIVER SUPPORT AND ESTROGEN DETOXIFICATION

- DIM (Diindolylmethane): Estroblock Pro Triple Strength
- Milk Thistle (I recommend HealthForce Superfoods Liver Rescue) paired with Holy Basil
- Magic Sea Moss by SOL Solutions (contains sea moss, bladderwrack, dandelion)
- Calcium D-Glucarate
- N-acetyl Cysteine
- Alpha Lipoic Acid
- Herbal Detox Support Teas: Milk Thistle, Dandelion, Burdock Root, Fennel, Licorice, Ginger

ANTI-INFLAMMATORY SUPPORT

- ☐ Bacopa Monnieri
- ☐ Turmeric Curcumin (with black pepper extract for absorption)
- ☐ SAM-e
- ☐ Shilajit
- ☐ Reishi
- ☐ CBD Oil

ANTI-STRESS AND HPA AXIS SUPPORTING

- ☐ Peony and Licorice (or plain licorice root)
- ☐ L-theanine
- ☐ Rhodiola
- ☐ American Ginseng
- ☐ Bacopa Monnieri
- ☐ Ashwagandha
- ☐ Holy Basil
- ☐ Lucuma
- ☐ Phosphatidylserine
- ☐ Cordyceps
- ☐ Schisandra Berry
- ☐ Astragalus
- ☐ Mucuna
- ☐ CBD Oil

DIGESTION, MICROBIOME AND GUT HEALTH

- ☐ Digestive Enzymes
- ☐ Probiotics
- ☐ L-glutamine
- ☐ Reishi
- ☐ CBD Oil
- ☐ Diatomaceous Earth
- ☐ Herbal Teas: Fennel, Ginger, Licorice, Peppermint

BLOOD SUGAR & INSULIN SUPPORT

- ☐ Berberine
- ☐ Inositol
- ☐ Holy Basil
- ☐ Chromium
- ☐ Alpha Lipoic Acid
- ☐ Cinnamon

FOR SLEEP AND INSOMNIA SUPPORT

- ☐ Ashwagandha
- ☐ Holy Basil
- ☐ Melatonin
- ☐ CALM Magnesium Tea
- ☐ CBD Oil
- ☐ Herbal Teas: Chamomile, Magnolia Bark, Valerian Root (can cause grogginess)
- ☐ Essential Oils: Lavender, Cedarwood, Chamomile, Vetiver, Sandalwood, Ylang Ylang

DEPRESSION AND ANXIETY SUPPORT

- [ ] St. John's Wort
- [ ] SAM-e (S-adenosylmethionine)
- [ ] L-theanine
- [ ] Genius Joy (combines l-theanine, l-tyrosine, SAM-e, 5-HTP, Rhodiola)
- [ ] Reishi
- [ ] Holy Basil
- [ ] He Shou Wu
- [ ] Mucuna
- [ ] Lucuma
- [ ] CBD Oil

BRAIN SUPPORT, FOCUS & CONCENTRATION, COGNITION, MOOD ENHANCEMENT

- [ ] B-complex
- [ ] Bacopa Monnieri
- [ ] L-theanine
- [ ] Rhodiola
- [ ] Gotu Kola
- [ ] Lions Mane
- [ ] Eleuthero
- [ ] Saw Palmetto
- [ ] Cordyceps

BOOST FERTILITY

- [ ] Vitex (Chaste-Tree Berry)
- [ ] Ashwagandha
- [ ] Maca powder (the red variety)
- [ ] Myo-inositol
- [ ] DIM (Diindolylmethane - Estroblock Pro)
- [ ] Shatavari

LIBIDO SUPPORT

- [ ] Maca powder or capsules
- [ ] Cistanche
- [ ] Cordyceps
- [ ] Moringa
- [ ] Schisandra Berry

MENOPAUSE SYMPTOMS

- [ ] Dong Quai
- [ ] Black Cohosh
- [ ] Maca powder (the red variety)
- [ ] Red Clover
- [ ] Coenzyme Q10
- [ ] Caffeine and Soy Products

ACNE

- [ ] DIM (Diindolylmethane - Estroblock Pro)
- [ ] Holy Basil
- [ ] Milk Thistle
- [ ] Berberine
- [ ] Herbal Detox Support Teas: Milk Thistle, Dandelion, Burdock Root, Fennel, Licorice, Ginger

THE HAPPY HORMONE METHOD

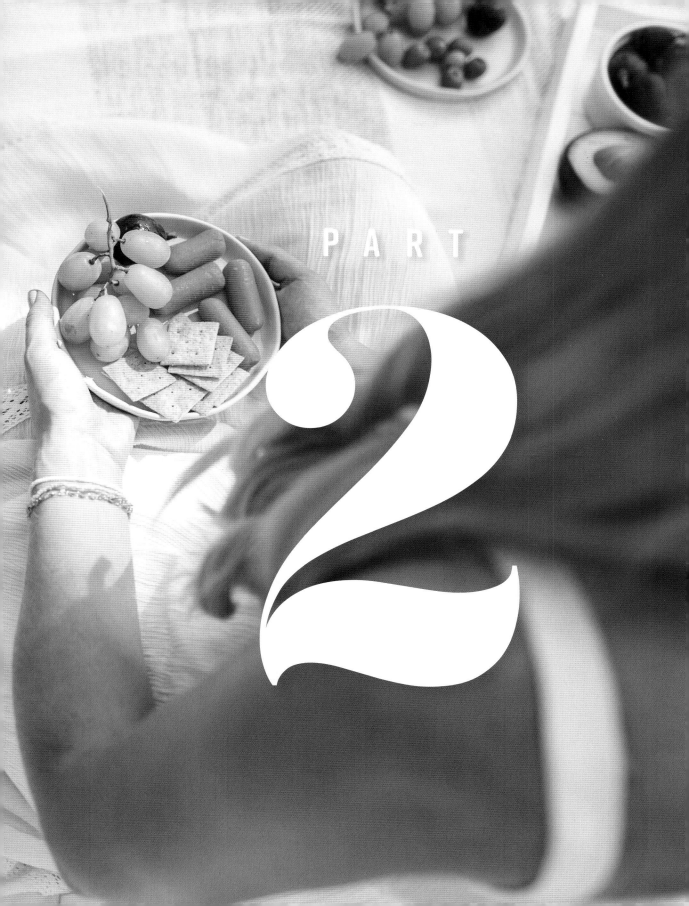

PART

2

CHAPTER

6

LIFESTYLE
ACTION STEPS

WELCOME TO THE HAPPY HORMONE METHOD. You are now equipped with the knowledge and understanding to begin your new lifestyle. In Part 1, you learned about the endocrine system and how internal and external factors affect hormone balance. Now you can put this knowledge into practice through the Happy Hormone Method and reap the incredible benefits of living, eating, and exercising with each phase of your cycle.

Before launching into the specifics of each cycle phase, it's important to set your body up for success using the following four lifestyle action steps. These are to be implemented *now* and *continuously* throughout the Happy Hormone Method. They are the pillars for bringing about natural hormone balance and optimal health. They build on each other, and each plays a part in supporting you for the long term.

THE LIFESTYLE ACTION STEPS ARE:

- ☐ Managing blood sugar, cortisol, and stress
- ☐ Removing endocrine disruptors
- ☐ Promoting digestion and elimination
- ☐ Harmonizing food and workouts

Your hormones won't become balanced overnight. It likely took years to throw off your hormone balance, so it will take time to put the pieces back together—3–6 months or longer. The Happy Hormone Method is a new way of living which incorporates a lot of change, but I wouldn't be here writing this book for you if I didn't whole-heartedly believe in this lifestyle.

I. MANAGING BLOOD SUGAR

Managing blood sugar is the most important hurdle when starting the Happy Hormone Method. If you don't get this action step right, your endocrine system won't have the chance to function at an optimal level.

Blood sugar (blood glucose) comes from the foods you eat and drink. Your brain relies on glucose for fuel, and your cells need it for energy. After every meal or beverage that you consume, your pancreas secretes a hormone called insulin into your bloodstream. Insulin tells your cells it's okay to use this glucose for energy. It then stores any extra glucose that your body doesn't immediately need in your liver and cells, for future use. When blood sugar gets low, such as in between meals or during exercise, the glucose is released. But if the extra glucose never gets used up, then it gets stored as fat.

HIGH BLOOD SUGAR

Major blood sugar problems arise when you consume inflammatory, processed foods, and refined sugars. While some of these may provide a spike of quick energy, they also cause a quick blood sugar drop which leaves you feeling fatigued, irritated, and craving more sugar, often leading to weight gain. These high-glycemic foods include things like donuts, sugary cereals, white or wheat toast, soda with artificial sweeteners, fruit juices which are high in sugar and loaded with empty calories, low-calorie "diet" foods, chips, cookies, and candy. Any of these foods will spike your blood glucose to high levels.

The endocrine system relies on blood sugar stability. Your body interprets mismanaged blood sugar as internal stress and in turn, signals your adrenal glands to release cortisol and adrenaline. From there, all your body can focus on is stabilizing your blood sugar levels, and you will feel the rollercoaster effects for the rest of the day. Having consistent, elevated blood glucose levels leads to insulin resistance, which can lead to prediabetes and type 2 diabetes.

LOW BLOOD SUGAR

On the other hand, when you eat too many carbs, the opposite can happen: low blood sugar (or hypoglycemia). After you consume an excess of carbs, the pancreas can pump out too much insulin. This extra insulin uses up too much of the glucose, and you are back at square one with low blood sugar and feeling hungry again. I think we've all experienced this: eating a big meal, feeling hungry an hour later and wondering why. In addition to eating too many carbs, low blood sugar can result from skipping meals, restricting certain food groups, and not eating enough calories.

Because your brain runs on glucose, it's hard to stay focused when your blood sugar is low. The best thing to do is to eat food that gradually raises your blood sugar, rather than high-glycemic food which will cause a spike and then a crash. Keeping blood sugar stable will help your pancreas release insulin only in the amounts it needs. When your blood sugar is balanced, you'll feel energized, upbeat, focused, and productive. It's your job to pay attention to your blood sugar throughout the entire day and respond before it gets too low, with foods that won't spike your blood sugar.

Managing blood sugar requires effort and planning. It doesn't happen by chance, it happens from making conscious choices at every meal—from the time you wake up until your head hits the pillow at night. But once you understand how to eat to stabilize blood sugar and recognize signs of an imbalance, you'll be on the right track.

SIGNS OF BLOOD SUGAR IMBALANCE

- ☐ Intense sugar and carb cravings
- ☐ Difficulty losing weight
- ☐ Belly fat
- ☐ Brain fog
- ☐ Jittery
- ☐ Poor memory
- ☐ Feeling hangry, woozy, or jittery if you miss a meal
- ☐ Fatigue after eating
- ☐ Irritability

HOW TO KEEP YOUR BLOOD SUGAR STABLE

The following techniques probably appear obvious and easy enough to manage, but sometimes it takes a closer look into what we are eating (not just what we think we're eating) to realize the areas in which we can improve. Hidden sugar is everywhere, in everything. All in all, it's best to limit your sugar intake altogether, plus it's nice to live a life that isn't controlled by sugar cravings.

AVOID PROCESSED, INFLAMMATORY FOODS

Stick to low-glycemic foods like veggies, leafy greens, legumes, nuts, and seeds, and low-sugar fruits (berries, cherries, pears, apricots, plums, and apples are best for this). If you want a fruit that's higher in sugar, pair it with a fat source to avoid blood sugar spikes, like a banana with peanut butter, or mango with coconut.

The top inflammatory foods to avoid include refined sugar, artificial sweeteners, alcohol, wheat, gluten, dairy products, and processed vegetable oils (canola oil, corn oil, soybean oil, sunflower oil, cottonseed oil, and safflower oil).

BALANCE MEALS WITH FIBER, HEALTHY FAT AND COMPLEX CARBS

Instead of eliminating all carbohydrates, make sure carbs or sugars are from whole foods (like fruit, starchy veggies, or whole grains) and balance them with the other macronutrients. Include a source of protein, fiber, and healthy fat with all of your meals. Doing this will slow the absorption of sugar into the bloodstream and prevent blood sugar spikes or drops.

For more on macronutrients, see chapter 4 on page 67.

USE NATURAL SWEETENERS AND WHITE FLOUR ALTERNATIVES

You may not even realize how much sugar you consume until you start paying more attention to every single thing you eat. Make sure to look at the labels.

I encourage you to switch to natural sugar alternatives derived from plants or fruit, instead of relying on refined sugars.

Remove any artificial sweeteners from your diet immediately. They hinder sugar metabolism, damage intestinal bacteria, and alter how your body processes fat which can cause weight gain and an increased risk for obesity and diabetes.

NATURAL SUGAR-FREE SWEETENERS (THESE WILL NOT SPIKE YOUR BLOOD SUGAR)

- ☐ Monk fruit granulated sweetener (I prefer the Lakanto brand)
- ☐ Medjool dates (they are whole foods after all)
- ☐ Stevia liquid drops (I prefer the flavored Sweet Leaf Sweet Drops)
- ☐ ChocZero sugar-free syrup
- ☐ Coconut sugar and maple syrup (I use these on special occasions for baking or desserts)

White flour is refined, processed, and highly inflammatory. Because it is stripped of all nutritional value, it spikes your blood sugar. The vitamins and minerals they add to enriched white flour are not bioavailable to us, meaning our bodies can't utilize them, so the added nutrients are pointless. Enriched or refined white flour is mostly used in junk foods like cookies, cakes, bread, cereals, pasta, donuts, pretzels, chips, muffins, and more.

Instead of baking or eating foods with white flour, try experimenting with almond flour, chickpea flour, TigerNut flour, gluten-free oat flour, buckwheat flour, or coconut flour, as they are naturally gluten-free and make for great alternatives in your cooking or baking.

Cinnamon

Cinnamon helps to balance blood sugar and tastes delicious in all types of dishes. I sprinkle it on smoothies, coffee, energy balls, apples, roasted sweet potatoes, baked goods, and more.

EAT WHEN YOU FEEL HUNGRY

A general guideline is to eat your first meal within 90 minutes of waking, but because I eat intuitively, I like to recommend having your first meal when you feel hungry (instead of forcing down food). I typically eat my first meal around 10 a.m., sometimes earlier or later—it just depends on how I feel. I don't beat myself up over when I'm hungry because every day is different. This doesn't mean you should wait until 10 a.m. to eat. It means making the connection to when you feel hungry and then feeding your body a balanced meal instead of skipping it or holding off until you feel ravenous and ready to binge everything in sight. Listening is how to build trust and intuition with your body, and the more you practice, the louder those food and hunger cues become.

Finding an eating routine that works intuitively for you is the only way you can tune into what your body needs. I won't say you need to eat three large meals per day at a specific time with snacks every two hours in between, or six small meals spaced throughout the day with no snacking. Unless you're an Olympic athlete on a strict diet plan, too many rules create a lot of food noise and make us constantly think about eating, even when we aren't hungry. What I recommend is getting your calories in whatever way works for you, whether from three large meals, with or without snacks, or six small meals. I think you'll find that when you start eating balanced meals with adequate fiber that won't spike your blood sugar, you'll experience fewer cravings and feel satisfied for longer periods. This may nudge you toward three larger meals each day, with or without snacks. This is how following the Happy Hormone Method unfolded for me.

What I don't recommend is starting your day with just coffee, as this will spike your blood sugar and set up your day to be full of cravings. Adding some fat and protein will alleviate a spike, but you'll have to experiment because metabolism and hunger fluctuate throughout each phase. That's why following your intuition is your best guiding light.

Hydrate First

It's easy to confuse dehydration with hunger. To prevent this, drink 16-32 ounces of filtered water first thing in the morning (preferably room-temperature or warm—no ice), and then 30 minutes before each meal. This will help you gauge how hungry you are, and keep you hydrated throughout the day.

HOW DO YOU KNOW HOW MUCH WATER YOU NEED? You should be drinking at least half of your body weight in ounces per day. So, if you weigh 140 pounds, you should be drinking 70 ounces of water, spread throughout the day.

To replenish electrolytes and mineral stores, see my "Sticky Water" recipe in the Happy Hormone Sips section on page 215.

ELIMINATE SWEET BEVERAGES AND LIMIT ALCOHOL

Drinking fruit juice is like drinking liquid sugar because there is nothing (like fiber, protein, or fat) to slow down its release into the bloodstream. Many "healthy" beverages have almost as much sugar as a can of cola, which contains 39 grams of sugar (that equates to about ten teaspoons of table sugar). An 8-ounce glass of orange juice has 18–24 grams of sugar, and a typical "energy" drink has 32 grams. Certain pasteurized green juices have upwards of 28 grams per serving. Always read labels and ingredient lists to check the sugar content. Stick with water, water infused with lemon, cucumber or mint, sparkling mineral water, or herbal tea.

Alcohol can also spike your blood sugar. It's also hard on your liver, and when balancing hormones, your liver needs to be healthy and functioning optimally. Try to cut back on your alcohol consumption as much as possible, limited to one or two times per week, or 2–3 drinks per week. Stick with low sugar options like vodka, tequila, dry red wine, or prosecco, and stay away from sugary mixers. Instead, mix with soda water, fresh lemon or lime, or kombucha.

Better yet, consider a mocktail, like my Ginger Lime Mocktail recipe in the Happy Hormone Sips section on page 217!

LIMIT CAFFEINE

Limit your caffeine as much as possible. If you must drink coffee, limit it to one cup per day. If drinking on an empty stomach, add one tablespoon of MCT oil or coconut oil to slow the release of caffeine and prevent a blood sugar rollercoaster. It's best to pair caffeine with a balanced meal.

EXERCISE 4-5 TIMES PER WEEK

Exercising lowers blood sugar levels by improving glucose metabolism. It helps your body clear sugar out of the bloodstream and into your muscles and tissues for fuel, instead of being stored as fat. Use your intuition and follow the exercise recommendations for each cycle phase.

MANAGE CORTISOL AND STRESS

Cortisol helps manage internal and external stressors. This means it helps regulate blood sugar levels, but as you learned earlier, it also helps you manage stress from the external world. Managing blood sugar ties into regulating cortisol and stress because they are often intertwined. High cortisol can lead to binging on sugary, processed foods that may feel comforting for a short time but will ultimately spike your blood sugar. When you are on the high blood sugar rollercoaster, every little stressor or issue you encounter throughout the day is amplified, which can stress you out even more. It becomes a vicious cycle.

To lower and flush cortisol levels, you may consider establishing new ways of managing day-to-day stress, on top of eating the right foods to keep your blood sugar in balance.

STRESS REDUCTION TECHNIQUES

- ☐ Say no more often without feeling guilty, or feeling like you have to explain yourself
- ☐ Surround yourself with people who bring you up rather than put you down
- ☐ Adopt a meditation practice
- ☐ Practice deep breathing exercises
- ☐ Seek therapy for an outside, unbiased perspective to manage your stress
- ☐ Spend more time in nature
- ☐ Do phase-appropriate exercises
- ☐ Eliminate/limit caffeine and/or stimulant use
- ☐ Turn your phone off or spend less time on it
- ☐ Get enough high-quality rest
- ☐ Take an Epsom salt bath
- ☐ Diffuse relaxing essential oils
- ☐ Get more facials or massages
- ☐ Read for fun or to relax
- ☐ Schedule self-care in your daily routine and do whatever self care means to you
- ☐ Have regular orgasms
- ☐ Snuggle with your pet or cuddle with your partner
- ☐ Do nothing at all, and truly relax

Many herbs and adaptogens can help your body adapt to stress better, lower cortisol levels, and help get you through stressful times. See my Anti-Stress and HPA Axis Supporting Supplements on page 90.

2. REMOVING ENDOCRINE DISRUPTORS

The world is full of endocrine disruptors, and it takes conscious effort to avoid or minimize exposure to these chemicals. This is a critical part of the Happy Hormone Method because, as you learned earlier in chapter 2, endocrine-disrupting chemicals (also known as EDC's) interfere with hormone action and mimic certain hormones, which trick your system into thinking it has to pump out more of one hormone and less of another. They can lead to all kinds of symptoms, from estrogen-related hormonal conditions such as PCOS, endometriosis, fibroids, and cysts, to unexplained headaches and extreme fatigue.

GUIDELINES FOR CREATING A NON-TOXIC HOME

You don't have to do it all at once, but over time, you can begin to replace your cleaning supplies, skin care, makeup, nail polish, and other products with non-toxic, healthier options. When your moisturizer or mascara runs out, try a new hormone-friendly, non-toxic brand. The point is to be more aware of what you are buying, using, cleaning with, and applying to your skin and hair.

FOOD & WATER

- Avoid pesticides, herbicides, and fungicides by choosing organic, locally-grown, and seasonal foods whenever possible. Helpful resources are the *Dirty Dozen* and *Clean Fifteen* lists (refer to https://www.ewg.org/).
- Wash all produce before eating. I recommend using a natural fruit and veggie wash.
- Consider an activated carbon water filter, for your at-home drinking water to filter out contaminants like pathogenic bacteria, viruses, chloramine, trihalomethanes, pharmaceuticals, pesticides, heavy metals, etc.
- Use a chlorine filter on shower heads.
- Buy BPA-free packaged and canned goods.

DIY Fruit and Veggie Wash

2 tablespoons distilled white vinegar + 2 tablespoons lemon juice + 1 cup tap water

Combine in a spray bottle and shake well before using.
Spray on your produce, scrub, and rinse.

PLASTICS

☐ Reduce plastic use as much as possible.

☐ Bring reusable cloth bags for groceries and shopping to avoid plastic grocery bags. Also, consider reusable cloth produce bags.

☐ Say no to plastic straws or consider bringing your own reusable straw when dining out.

☐ Avoid microwaving food in plastic containers.

☐ Avoid using plastic wrap and baggies when storing or wrapping food. Use reusable food wraps instead. I also love reusable, dishwasher-safe silicone bags in lieu of single use plastic bags.

☐ Use glass or ceramic containers for food storage. I also love storing food in mason jars.

☐ Drink out of glass containers only. Consider a reusable glass water bottle to bring out with you, instead of buying cases of plastic water bottles.

HOME AND CLEANING SUPPLIES

☐ Use non-toxic, chemical-free, biodegradable, household cleaning products, laundry detergent, fabric softener, dish soap, dish detergent, and hand soap (I love the products from Seventh Generation, Branch Basics, Meyers, and Raw Sugar).

☐ Clean with safe, common, household ingredients like baking soda, white vinegar, natural soap, lemons, and essential oils.

☐ Use clean candle brands (like Element, Lite + Cycle or Keap), or use an essential oil diffuser instead. I love freshening up the kitchen after cooking by diffusing lemon essential oil.

☐ Avoid nonstick pots and pans and consider carbon steel, stainless steel, ceramic, or copper. Or choose ceramic nonstick pans that are free of PFAS, PFOA, lead, and cadmium.

☐ Add houseplants to a few rooms in your home. The soil bacteria helps to reduce the volatile organic compounds (like formaldehyde) in the air.

☐ Consider switching to "green" dry cleaners that don't use perchloroethylene or "perc" in their dry cleaning services.

☐ Take off your shoes at the front door to avoid tracking in lead, dust, pesticides, and bacteria.

☐ Vacuum your house regularly using a HEPA filter. This filters out many of the chemicals from the dust in your home, like fire retardants, phthalates, and pesticides.

Top Ingredients to Avoid in Cleaning Products

- 2-Bromo-2-Nitropropane-1,3-Diol
- Alkyl Dimethyl Benzyl Ammonium Chloride
- Alkyl Dimethyl Ethylbenzyl Ammonium Chloride
- Didecyldimethylammonium Chloride
- Diethanolamine
- Dioctyl Dimethyl Ammonium Chloride
- Distearyldimonium Chloride
- DMDM Hydantoin
- Ethanolamine
- Formaldehyde
- Glutaral
- Monoethanolamine Citrate
- Quaternium-15
- Quaternium-24
- Sodium Hypochlorite (Bleach)
- Sulfuric Acid
- Triethanolamine

BEAUTY AND COSMETIC PRODUCTS

- ☐ Read your cosmetic ingredient labels and avoid harmful ingredients (see below).

- ☐ Check products (I like using EWG's Skin Deep website or Think Dirty app) to see where brands and products rank and their toxicity score.

- ☐ Choose clean beauty brands (see a list of my favorite brands for skin care, hair care, makeup, toothpaste, deodorant, sunscreen, nail polish, and all things beauty on page 40).

- ☐ Shop the clean beauty online stores like *Credo Beauty, CAP Beauty, The Detox Market,* and *Beauty Counter.*

- ☐ Switch to a more natural spa or salon for your beauty, hair, and skin treatments.

- ☐ Use naturally-derived fragrances from plants or essential oils, instead of artificial fragrances.

- ☐ Avoid toxic menstrual products and tampons (see my natural menstrual product recommendations on page 128).

- ☐ Avoid hand sanitizers (or opt for natural options from Dr. Bronner's, Meyers, or EO).

Top Ingredients to Avoid in Beauty Products

- Benzalkonium Chloride
- BHA/BHT
- Butyl Alcohol
- Butylatedhydroxy Anisole
- Butylated Hydroxytoluene
- Diazolidinyl Urea
- Disodium EDTA
- DMDM Hydantoin
- Ethanol
- Ethylenediaminetetraacetic acid (EDTA)
- Ethylene Glycol
- Ethanolamines (MEA/DEA/TEA)
- Formaldehyde
- Fragrance
- Hydroquinone
- Imidazolidinyl Urea
- Lithium Chloride
- Methylisothiazolinone
- Methylene Chloride
- Oxybenzone
- PABA (Para-aminobenzoic acid)
- Parabens (methyl-, isobutyl-, propyl-)
- PEG (and anything containing ceteareth, xynol and oleth)
- Petrochemicals (like mineral oil, petroleum jelly, propylene glycol, paraffin)
- Phthalates (DBP, DEHP, DEP)
- Phenoxyethanol
- Polyethylene glycol
- Poly Quaternium (7, 10, 11, 15)
- Retinyl palmitate
- Retinol
- Sodium Lauryl Sulfate
- Sodium Laureth Sulfate (SLS and SLES)
- Stearalkonium chloride
- Talc
- Toulene
- Triclosan
- Triclocarban
- Urea
- VOC's (volatile organic compounds)

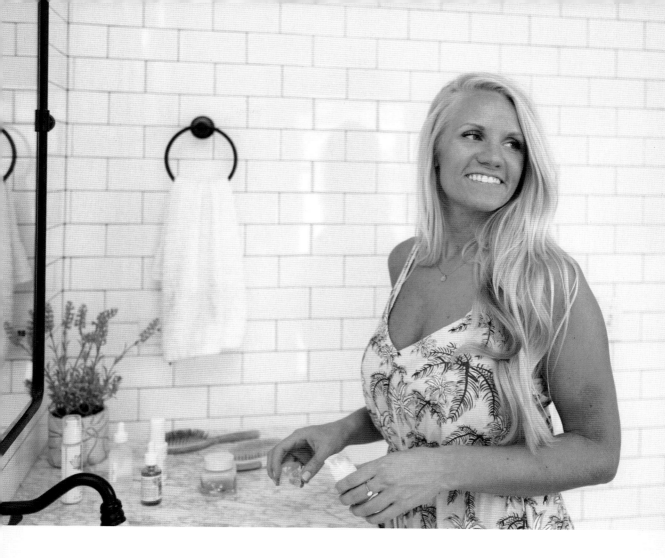

AT WORK AND PUBLIC PLACES

- ☐ Salons, housekeeping services, and golf courses are some of the highest endocrine-disrupting occupations, due to the products used and chemicals sprayed.

- ☐ Say *no* to paper receipts as they are full of highly absorbable phenol chemicals like BPA and BPS (Bisphenol A and Bisphenol S), and they waste paper.

- ☐ Be aware of toxic fumes from copiers, printers, carpets, construction sites, and building materials.

- ☐ Avoid drinking fountain water and bring filtered water in a reusable bottle.

- ☐ Avoid heating your work lunch in plastic in the microwave. Use glass instead and bring your own silverware.

3. SUPPORTING DIGESTION AND ELIMINATION

Many things can overburden the liver and slow down elimination pathways. These include environmental toxins, endocrine disruptors, physical and emotional stress, travel, lack of sleep, poor diet, and unhealthy gut bacteria. All of these can make it hard for your liver to metabolize estrogen. This build-up of estrogen can interrupt your natural hormonal ecosystem and produce various signs and symptoms of estrogen dominance. You can't have healthy periods with an unhealthy microbiome, so the key is to establish regular bowel movements and maintain healthy intestinal flora. There are a few ways to do this.

DETOX & NOURISH YOUR LIVER

- [ ] Consume at least 25 grams of fiber per day (see my High Fiber Happy Hormone Foods on page 71).

- [ ] Eat 1–2 brazil nuts per day for selenium.

- [ ] Take liver-supporting herbs and supplements (see page 89).

- [ ] Drink herbal detox-supporting teas such as dandelion, burdock root, fennel, licorice, or ginger.

- [ ] Always drink and cook with filtered water instead of tap.

TREAT YOUR MICROBIOME

Optimizing your gut flora is essential for hormone health and a well-functioning immune system, which in turn helps fight chronic inflammation and promotes elimination of estrogen. After taking all the steps to balance your blood sugar and care for your liver, work to nourish your gut. In addition to taking a daily probiotic (see page 87), try the following.

- [ ] Eat fermented vegetables and traditionally cultured foods. These will help replenish your gut with beneficial bacteria and include non-dairy yogurt (unsweetened or plain), sauerkraut, kimchi, olives, miso, tempeh, natto, and pickles.

- [ ] Take a digestive enzyme before meals to assist with absorption of nutrients from your food (I prefer the Renew Life Plant Based Enzymes) or take a shot of apple cider vinegar before eating.

- [ ] Consider L-glutamine for healing your intestinal lining and supporting overall gut health, especially if you experience IBS symptoms. L-glutamine is an essential amino acid that works to protect the mucous membranes of your intestines and esophagus. It boosts immune cell activity and soothes intestinal lining.

4. MATCH YOUR FOOD AND WORKOUTS

The Food:

At the center of the Happy Hormone Method lies the specific foods you should focus on throughout each cycle phase to nutritionally support your fluctuating hormones and micronutrient needs. Certain foods can support your rising estrogen in the menstrual and follicular phases, and then support proper estrogen detoxification in the ovulatory and luteal phases so that progesterone has time to shine. You might be used to this way of eating, or it may feel daunting and new. Either way, I'm here to guide you through it. It's not about being perfect, but more so realizing how your daily eating habits can bring the most significant improvements to your hormone health, simply by eating certain foods at different times in your cycle. As you will see, each phase has its own chapter with phase-specific food lists and recipes. These foods and recipes will guide your daily meals, snacks and even, desserts.

The Workouts:

Exercise is an integral part of the Happy Hormone Method. Just as you focus on different foods for each phase, you'll also harmonize workouts for each phase. It's about committing and connecting with your body and recognizing where you are. Doing this not only honors your energy levels, hormone ratios and how you feel in each phase, but it also offers a new perspective on how to treat your body throughout the month. This means putting the extra energy you have to good use in the first half of your cycle (follicular and ovulatory phases) and doing more bodyweight, restorative-type exercises in the second half (luteal and menstrual). As you read on about each phase, you will see that I list optimal workouts to honor your physical abilities, hormone levels, and energy.

It may take some getting used to but pushing through an intense workout while on your period can do more harm than good, as it's a better time for restorative exercise. Exercise is meant to burn off extra energy (when we have it) and make us feel good. It's not about pushing through strenuous workouts we hate when we're sluggish, off balance, or lacking in energy, just for the sake of crossing cardio off our to-do list.

CHAPTER

7

GET READY TO CYCLE

BEFORE YOU START SYNCING UP WITH THE PHASES OF YOUR CYCLE, this chapter focuses on a few final tips to keep in mind and help pull it all together to answer any remaining questions you may have. There are so many helpful tools for period, ovulation, and symptom tracking nowadays, which makes living with the Happy Hormone Method that much easier. You just have to experiment and find the tools that resonate with you.

START TRACKING YOUR CYCLE

For a rough idea of the phase you're in, enter your most recent period data (day and length of period) into a period tracking app (see app recommendations), for a rough estimate of where you are in your cycle. If you don't know exactly when your last period was, a rough guess will do. We all have to start somewhere, and this will be yours.

It's important to note that learning the signs and symptoms of each phase takes months, especially if you are new to period tracking and your cycle is irregular. It's not about being perfect right away, but about learning the ebbs and flows of your cycle, how you feel as it changes, and getting more in tune with your body. Be patient. Continue tracking signs and symptoms from here on out, such as: what day you get your period, when it stops, if and when you notice cervical fluid throughout the month, what types of symptoms you experience, signs of ovulation (more on this in the Ovulatory phase chapter, page 172) so the app—and you—can get to know your cycle. Tracking is a wonderful way to connect to your body and learn the rhythms of your cycle.

PERIOD APPS AND FERTILITY TRACKING TOOLS

There are so many great period and fertility tracking apps and tools. Most apps are free, and some are for period tracking only, while others go more in-depth with options for tracking ovulation, cervical mucus, PMS symptoms, sexual activity and more. You can go even further with upgraded thermometers for fertility monitoring, such as the Daysy Fertility Monitor or the Wink by Kindara that take precise morning oral temperatures and keep track of your readings by syncing your data to the corresponding app.

The Daysy determines your fertile and infertile days using a color system based on your daily temperature, with 99.4% accuracy. It learns the rhythm of your body over the span of 2–3 cycles. Your data then syncs up with the DaysyView app. I use the Daysy and set it on top of my phone before bed so that I see it as soon as I wake up, which reminds me to take my temperature. I love how it tells me immediately if the day is either red (fertile), yellow (caution), or green (infertile). The Wink works in essentially the same way; it just depends on which you prefer.

Another option is the Ava bracelet, which detects your five most fertile days of each cycle for those who are trying to conceive or want to avoid pregnancy. It also includes insights about your sleep, stress, and resting heart rate.

Another bonus is being able to download your data and bring it to your doctor for further analyzing in relation to hormonal problems such as PCOS or thyroid conditions.

PERIOD AND CYCLE TRACKING APPS: *Kindara, MyFLO tracker, Flo, Clue, Glow, Life, Eve, Natural Cycles, My Cycles, Ovia, and Ferdy.*

CHARTING YOUR BASAL BODY TEMPERATURE (BBT)

If these upgraded thermometers are out of your price range, using a basal body thermometer and charting your temperature throughout your cycle works just fine, too. You can buy a basal body thermometer at any drugstore or online. To obtain a precise reading, you must take your temperature before sitting up or getting out of bed—literally as soon as you wake up.

The temperature charting method is quick, easy, and accurate. A noticeable temperature rise happens right after ovulation because progesterone raises your core body temperature. If you're lucky, you may notice a sharp drop in temperature on the day of ovulation. The follicular and ovulatory phases consist of lower temperature readings, while the luteal and menstrual phases are higher. A basal body thermometer measures more sensitively with two decimal points (example: 97.67 instead of 97.6) giving you a precise prediction into whether or not you've ovulated this cycle.

When you see at least three higher-than-average readings in a row, it's a great indication that ovulation occurred on the day before your first high temperature. There are many example charts of this online. At the end of your luteal phase, you will notice a temperature drop, meaning you will probably get your period that day. If it remains high, this could be a sign of pregnancy. BBT charting will not help you predict ovulation or tell you when you are fertile, but it can be used to confirm that ovulation did happen. Regular ovulation is important for many reasons that we'll discuss in chapter 10.

BEGIN SYNCING YOUR FOOD TO EACH PHASE

Depending on where you are in your cycle, start to focus on each phase-specific chapter for food, workouts and everything in between. You may be wondering, how am I going to remember what foods to eat and when? I thought the same things in the beginning, but I created the Happy Hormone Method to make it easy for you. The following chapters walk you through what you need to remember for every phase of your cycle, including some of my favorite recipes.

And don't expect to be perfect. Life, parties, and vacations happen, but you can always come right back. There are weeks when eating something quick matters more to me than eating something phase-friendly, but that doesn't mean I throw it all out the window. I make choices at every single meal. So maybe all I can manage that day is a phase-friendly breakfast and snack, and that's fine. But I'm always striving to eat foods that make my hormones happy because when my hormones are happy, I'm happy.

Remember, you won't see significant changes overnight, but in 2-3 months, you should begin to notice significant improvements to your hormone balance and cycle. Give your body time to balance itself out, and don't give up.

CONSIDER EXAMS AND TESTING

Are you up to date with your OB-GYN exams to rule out obvious problems? After three months of following this plan, consider making an appointment for a full hormone, thyroid, and blood panel, to see where you are and gain some peace of mind. *Refer to the Labs and Hormone Testing Options on pages 32–35.*

This will allow you to dig deeper and see what additional herbs or supplements you can introduce. It may be especially helpful to work with a naturopath or holistic doctor as they are usually more open to herbs and treatment options, and they'll also help you understand your lab results. I don't recommend testing before the three-month mark because levels will usually improve, and you'll likely want another test.

After the first three months, I recommend testing every 6–12 months.

START A HAPPY HORMONE JOURNAL

Finally, I suggest picking out a special journal for taking notes throughout each phase. I will let you know what you need to be aware of and what things you may want to track, but ultimately, your hormone journal will help you get to know your cycle on a more intimate level. This helps you understand what to prepare for based on the previous month, so you can make plans and set goals accordingly. Keeping a record of symptoms, energy levels, moods, feelings, and what you may have changed when it comes to eating, exercise, or supplementation. You'll be aware of how your skin looks, the color of your period, of what you want to improve or do better with next month, and anything else relevant to your cycle.

Sometimes it's hard to notice patterns when they are spaced weeks apart. Journaling helps keep us aware and accountable, and shows what might need work. You may also notice how your moods and feelings can govern what you feel like doing, thanks to your fluctuating hormones. My moods are like clockwork, and I never connected the dots to hormones until I learned about the phases—even my partner can recognize what phase I'm in based on my moodiness or chattiness (he mispronounces most of the phases, but it's cute that he tries to understand where I'm at). Once you learn the waves of your cycle, it can be fun to include your partner and is somewhat enlightening for them.

For me, the journaling process feels therapeutic and also helps me remember what was going on three months ago that may be affecting my cycle this month (refer to the Hundred-Day Journey on page 129). Having a hormone journal opens up the lines of communication between mind and body and offers a chance to become more in tune with your hormonal shifts.

Happy Hormone
FAQS

Lastly, here are some answers to the most common questions I receive about living in harmony with your cycle:

CAN I USE THIS PLAN AND COME UP WITH MY OWN RECIPES, TOO?

Yes! This plan is meant to take the guesswork out of coming up with healthy, phase-appropriate, plant-based recipes. It's great if you can incorporate your ideas, too. For each phase, feel free to combine any of the foods on the food chart. I do this all the time (if you do create your own recipe, please share it and tag me on social media because I'd love to see it). You will soon be an expert in knowing what your body wants and when. The recipe possibilities are endless.

I WANT TO FOLLOW THE HAPPY HORMONE METHOD, BUT AM I REQUIRED TO EAT THE RECOMMENDED FOODS 100% OF THE TIME?

It took about six months for me to get the hang of eating with my hormonal fluctuations. In the beginning, I was not hormonally balanced so understanding the phase-specific foods and when to integrate them took time, as my body started to readjust. I began by incorporating just a few phase-appropriate foods at a time (I also had nothing to follow). I know it's impossible to eat only the recommended foods 100% of the time.

While the majority of the foods you eat should be phase-appropriate, it's important to be realistic. Do the best you can by aiming for 70% or more of phase-appropriate foods. Also, prepare the recommended foods in a way that makes you happy. If a cold green salad doesn't sound appetizing in the dead of winter during your ovulatory phase, add lightly steamed veggies or grains and make it more appealing to your palate. There are different ways to adapt cooking methods that align with each season while still eating the recommended foods for each phase.

WHAT HAPPENS IF I EAT FOOD THAT'S MEANT FOR A DIFFERENT PHASE?

No worries. It's okay if a portion of the food you're eating is meant for a different phase, as long as the majority of food is specific to the phase you're in. If you eat something on the protocol for the luteal phase but are in the follicular phase, nothing bad will happen. But your hormones are better supported with the macro and micronutrients from the follicular foods. I created this plan in line with what we tend to crave. The first half of your cycle (follicular and ovulatory) includes more fresh, raw and energizing foods, while the second half (luteal and menstrual phases) includes more comforting and grounding foods. For the most part, the food should appeal to your tastes in each phase.

HOW SHOULD I HANDLE PEOPLE WHO DON'T SUPPORT OR UNDERSTAND THE HAPPY HORMONE METHOD?

Living and eating in cyclical harmony with your hormone fluctuations is new and exciting, but you can't expect everyone to understand. People don't like change, especially when it comes to eating habits. Instead of worrying about it, stay in your lane and focus on what you want and how you want to feel. Mention that you're trying a new way of eating to feel better and increase your energy levels. No one can argue with that.

Remember, this is about your body, your journey, and the outcomes you desire. You don't even have to tell your partner or family unless you think they would find it interesting. Feel free to keep it to yourself until you feel comfortable. If you are cooking for your family or partner, all of the foods are healthy, and there's no reason they can't enjoy the recipes along with you.

Do share it with the women in your life, because this may be just the kind of plan they need. It helps to bounce ideas off of each other, share knowledge, and talk about the phases you're in. You can always come to me, too.

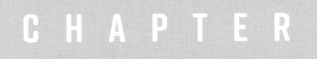

CHAPTER

8

THE FOUR
PHASES

IMILAR TO THE LUNAR MOON CYCLE AND THE FOUR SEASONS, your menstrual cycle has four unique phases: menstrual, follicular, ovulatory, and luteal. Just like winter, spring, summer, and autumn, your body transitions through four phases about every 28–30 days, on average. Each phase invites a unique set of hormonal, physical, emotional, and psychological gifts. When we understand these changes and eat, work, love, and play according to our natural flow, we get better at working with our feminine power rather than against it.

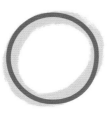 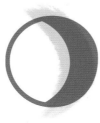  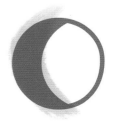

Menstrual
New Moon
Winter

Follicular
Waxing Moon
Spring

Ovulatory
Full Moon
Summer

Luteal
Waning Moon
Autumn

Note: If you take any form of hormonal birth control, you are not experiencing the four-cycle changes.

It's important to embrace and honor the changes throughout your cycle, but I find that most women don't even know the four distinct phases. They may be most familiar with the menstrual and ovulatory phases but not the other two. I was the same way. Once I started tracking my cycle and living in harmony with my hormones, I felt more connected to my body than ever before, which helped me appreciate my lady parts for the first time. Instead of the usual resentment toward PMS and my period, my mindset shifted, and I grew to acknowledge the immense work my body performs every month. I found that by purely honoring each phase, my intuition—the inner voice coming from my gut that we all have—grew stronger and clearer and is now the shining light that guides my life.

Men are more capable of performing the same daily routines due to their 24-hour hormonal cycles, but because we fluctuate through 28-day cycles (on average), doing the same things every day is not biologically sensible or realistic. That's what the Happy Hormone Method is all about.

In the next four sections, you will learn the ebbs and flows of your monthly cycle—the very thing that makes you a woman. Incredible health insights lie within each phase. By harmonizing your life with each phase of your cycle, you can harness your strengths, help your body heal, lose weight if there is any to be lost, and create a desirable life.

For each phase, I cover the optimal foods, appropriate workouts, changes in your cervical mucus, whether it's a "wet" or "dry" phase, how your skin changes with each fluctuation, the best types of skincare products (including DIY face mask recipes), typical mood and energy levels, what you should be focusing on at work, how to best schedule your social life and most importantly, what the heck is going on with your hormones and endocrine system.

Specifically, each phase chapter includes the following topics:

☐ Your Hormones	☐ Skin
☐ Your Period	☐ DIY Face and Hair Mask Recipes
☐ Mood & Energy	☐ Beauty and Wellness Tips
☐ Exercise	☐ Nutrition
☐ Sex	☐ Food Chart
☐ Lubrication	☐ Recipes

LUNAR CYCLES: WHITE MOON VS. RED MOON CYCLES

Do you think it's a coincidence that the length of your menstrual cycle syncs with the length of the lunar moon cycle, which occurs every 29 days? Understanding the phases of the moon opens the pathway of connecting your female body with the cyclical nature of planet earth, which we could all use in our hectic, screen-focused lives. I find it incredibly grounding and comforting to know that I align with the cycles of nature.

It is thought that the moon phases influence women's cycles. The highest rates of ovulation and conception occur on the full moon or the day before. As you'll see, this correlates with the ovulatory phase which makes sense because that is when you are most fertile. During the new moon, ovulation and conception rates are much lower with an increase in the number of women who start menstruation. This common, traditional way of cycling is called the *White Moon Cycle* and is historically influenced by the increased amount of bright light from the full moon and sunlight.

Your cycle may be flip-flopped. Instead, you might ovulate with the new moon and menstruate with the full moon. This is known as the *Red Moon Cycle*. These women are thought to be healers, wise women, medicine women, or midwives. They can help menstruating women while they themselves are ovulating, giving them the energy and opportunity to care for and teach others.

It is thought that you will experience both the White Moon Cycle and Red Moon Cycle in your lifetime. Just one more reason to avoid hormonal birth control and instead, go with the flow.

ALIGN YOUR CYCLE WITH THE MOON

As long as your cycle is consistent and healthy, that's all that matters. There's no need to worry if your cycle doesn't sync up with the moon. But if you feel intrigued, there are some steps you can take to gently shift your body to align with the moon cycle.

MAKE FRIENDS WITH THE MOON

The best way to get to know lunar cycles is to tune into the moon and find it in the sky every night. Better yet, go on an evening walk, especially during the full moon. Observe and appreciate the moon's fluctuations. This will fuel your connection and help your body adjust. If you live in a city or are unable to connect with the moon at night, then download a moon app on your phone (like My Moontime, Full Moon Phase or Moon Phase Calendar), or hang a moon phase calendar and have a moment with the moon every day.

REGULATE YOUR SLEEP

Get your circadian rhythm and sleep-wake cycle on track. Stay off of your phone and computer a couple of hours before bed to prevent the artificial blue light from interrupting your ability to fall asleep, or get blue light blocking glasses (my favorites are from Pixel Eyewear). Get to bed earlier and wake up earlier. Make sure your living space is bright with natural light when you wake up and throughout the day. If you're outside during the day, take off your sunglasses as often as possible. At night, keep the lights in your living space soft and dim, so your body knows the distinction between day and night.

GET CLOSE TO NATURE

Ideally, get outside and walk in the grass, soil, or sand without your shoes on for 20-30 minutes per day, or as often as possible. The earth has a natural kind of electric charge, and our bodies get charged up and "grounded" when we connect this way. This practice is well-known as "earthing" or "grounding" and has been shown to normalize the body's biological rhythms and reduce stress while also lessening hormonal and menstrual symptoms. Open your windows as often as possible and let some natural air circulate. Listen and connect to the sounds outside. Take daily walks to fill your lungs with fresh air. Bring nature inside with houseplants that clean the air. *Depending on where you live, "grounding" may not be possible in the winter months, but you can still bundle up and get outside to help your body with the distinction of day versus night.*

Here's a hormonal cycle chart of your fluctuating hormones throughout the month. This will help you in the upcoming chapters! Remember, day one is the start of your menstrual cycle.

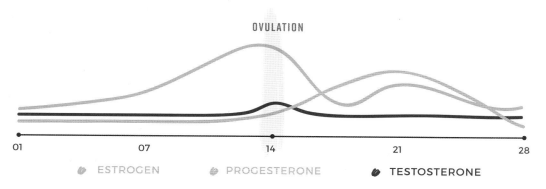

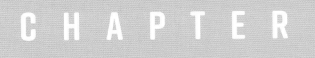

CHAPTER

9

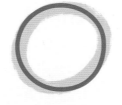

Phase One:

MENSTRUAL

Winter | New Moon

3-7 DAYS
BBT: 97.0 - 97.6

WINTER IN THE FEMALE BODY IS THOUGHT TO BE A TIME when the veil between your spirit and the earthly world is the thinnest. This means there is little distinction between intuition and logic, allowing you to access true inner wisdom. In ancient times, women used to separate from the men during their bleeding phase and gather in menstrual huts or tents to renew and tune into the spirit world.

When we explore winter in nature, it's a time to rest, turn inward and conserve energy. Some animals remove themselves from the world completely and transition into deep hibernation. Winter in the female body evokes a similar yearning to hibernate and rest because the body is busy shedding your endometrium (the innermost layer of your uterus), which may leave you feeling extra tired. This offers a chance to ease up on your schedule and slow down.

As we learned before, your period is naturally cleansing, releasing bacteria and excess iron from the body. It's also a time of emotional release and shedding what no longer serves you. During or right before your period, you may cry more easily. Take this time for internal healing and deep spiritual work. Periods are intricately intertwined with what's happening in our lives.

Day one of your period begins on the first day of heavy bleeding, not to be confused with any days of light spotting or brown-colored blood leading up to your first heavy day. Tracking your first heavy day will help determine the length of your cycle. It's the first piece of information you'll want to record in your hormone journal or period tracking app, along with any symptoms you may be experiencing, like the color of the blood each day (brown, bright red cranberry, dark crimson red, light pink), if there was spotting before your period or not, and how many days your period lasts.

The Changing Color of Your Period

At the start, period blood should be bright red and cranberry colored because it is flowing quickly. By the third or fourth day, your blood is flowing more slowly and may become darker and brown or even light pink, the more it is exposed to air. If you notice brown spotting *before* your first heavy day of bright red colored blood, that may be old blood from your previous cycle that has oxidized and may indicate low progesterone. Low levels may be linked to anovulatory cycles (cycles without ovulation).

If your period blood is very dark and almost eggplant purple in color, this may indicate high estrogen in proportion to progesterone. The opposite would be minimal, very light pink which could indicate low estrogen levels. This may happen after extreme dieting, adrenal fatigue, or nutrient deficiencies.

YOUR HORMONES

If you do not become pregnant, the corpus luteum (the empty follicle from which the egg was released that becomes an endocrine-secreting gland) stops producing progesterone and gets reabsorbed by the body. This drop in progesterone causes your uterus to contract, which is your body's way of eliminating the uterine lining and is also known as your period "bleed." On average, bleeding happens 12–14 days post-ovulation. After the bleeding phase, estrogen starts to rise which signals the hypothalamus to get your body ready for ovulation again.

THE BLEED

Your bleed should last anywhere from 3–7 days, starting moderately to heavy and gradually tapering off. The second day of bleeding may be the heaviest. You can expect 90% of total blood loss to take place within the first three days. It can be difficult to measure how much blood you're losing, and the amount will vary from woman to woman. Your period may range on the lighter side at 25 mL lost, or it may be on the heavy side at 80 mL, but the average is 35–50 mL (or 2–3 menstrual cups). There is no perfect amount.

HEAVY PERIODS: If you lose more than 80 mL every cycle and have to change your pad or tampon every hour, you are at higher risk for iron deficiency and may have an underlying imbalance (see page 199). It is worth getting your hormone and nutrient levels tested to see if there are underlying deficiencies. You may also want to get checked for fibroids, endometriosis, or adenomyosis by having your doctor do a full abdominal and transvaginal ultrasound. Diet and lifestyle factors are the primary culprits for estrogen–dominance. The Happy Hormone Method can help normalize heavy bleeding.

Note: Teenagers often experience heavy periods for the first couple of years of their cycle. This is normal and will usually subside with time as they mature to make more pro-gesterone, but can also be helped through diet and lifestyle. The birth control pill will not "fix" their heavy periods, but young endocrine systems can be supported with the Happy Hormone Method as they develop.

Natural Menstrual Products

Choose menstrual products with care; you use them almost every month of your adult life. The feminine care industry is not required to disclose ingredient lists, so choose products that aren't made with harmful chemicals, fragrances, gels, or additives. Here are my favorite products:

- **MENSTRUAL CUPS** Diva Cup, Lunette, Selena Cup
  Soft, reusable menstrual cups are made of medical-grade silicone and collect your blood instead of absorb it.

- **MENSTRUAL DISCS** Flex Disc, Soft Disc
  Disposable menstrual discs collect menstrual blood; they can be worn during sex since they don't block the vaginal canal.

- **ORGANIC COTTON TAMPONS & PADS** Cora, Seventh Generation, L.Organic, LOLA, Honest Company, Rael

- **REUSABLE PERIOD PADS AND LINERS** Glad Rags, Lunapads, Hesta, Charlie Banana

- **PERIOD UNDERWEAR** Thinx, Dear Kates, Modibodi, Harebrained, Lunapads, Knixteen, Panty Prop, Cute Fruit Undies
  Sustainable period underwear absorbs your period, traps moisture, and prevents leaks.

The Hundred-Day Journey

Here's something cool: it takes one hundred days for a follicle to mature from its beginning inactive state to mature enough for ovulation. A healthy period requires healthy follicles, so if you've had an unusual period count back three months. What may have happened during that time? Were you experiencing extra stress? Were you not eating as much or as healthy as usual? Were you not sleeping as much or maybe going out a little too often? What you do today will affect your cycle in three months. I love to bring this awareness to light because we often don't connect the dots that way. This is where tracking your cycle and keeping a hormone journal can be so beneficial—it helps you reflect, look for clues and patterns, and find clarity for the present day.

MOOD & ENERGY

Hormones are at their lowest levels during your period, which means you may naturally feel withdrawn, internal, and reflective. This is a time of introspection. Because your left and right brain hemispheres are communicating the most during this time, you feel the most in-tune with your gut, and whether or not anything needs to change moving forward. Consider this a chance to rewrite your life path. A common feeling during menstruation is discontent or uneasiness when life is not heading in the direction you desire, so you may feel an urge to end a relationship that is holding you back or a friendship that is no longer serving you. Any recurring thoughts, fears, or worries that come to the surface during this time, month after month, deserve your attention.

At work, you'll want to do the same: evaluate, assess, and pay attention to anything that could be improved. Then, in the follicular phase, you can make a plan and work on areas of change throughout the ovulatory and luteal phases. For now, your time is best spent reflecting and having cozy nights at home. Give yourself full permission to rest and recharge so your body can prepare for the weeks ahead.

EXERCISE

For this phase, think of soothing and restorative activities. Stretching, twisting, medicinal-type, and yin yoga are great options. Naps are welcomed especially in the first few days of your period. Toward the end of bleeding, energy will start to rise, so consider lighter exercise like walking, pilates, or whatever yoga feels good. *For an at-home workout video during this phase, I love the Floating Yoga School YouTube channel.*

SEX

Every woman has different desires during her period. You may want to abstain from sex and savor extra alone time to read a book or get pampered at the spa, or you may want to connect with your partner and have sex.

Even though your hormones are at their lowest levels during your period, you may experience an increase in libido. According to functional nutritionist Alisa Vitti, this is a structural phenomenon because your uterus is expanding with blood and pressing on nerve endings in your pelvic basin. When these nerve endings are stimulated, your brain may interpret it as if something were touching you there, which can put you in the mood.

LUBRICATION & CERVICAL MUCUS

If you are going to have sex on your period, you should know that although you are bleeding, menstruation is still considered a "dry phase" in your cycle. It may sound contradictory, but the types of cervical fluid differ throughout the month. While you may have discharge and blood, the kind of cervical fluid during this phase may not feel like ideal lubrication for sex (especially near the end of your period), which means you may want to supplement with some.

SKIN AND BEAUTY

During your period, you'll likely notice heightened skin sensitivity and more redness than usual from increased blood flow to your capillaries. Low estrogen levels may cause your skin to look dull and feel dry, making wrinkles, pores, or scarring appear more noticeable. I know it's not what you want to hear, but there are tips and tricks for amping up the glow. Focus on anti-inflammatory, calming, and soothing products that hydrate and put moisture back into the skin. As always, drink lots of filtered water.

DIY WINTER FACE MASK

Soothing Avocado Aloe Mask (for dull skin)

1 tablespoon mashed avocado

**1 tablespoon pure aloe vera gel
(with no added ingredients)**

**1 teaspoon oat flour (or
rolled oats)**

**1 teaspoon organic jojoba oil
(you can sub with rosehip oil or
pumpkin seed oil)**

Combine all ingredients in a small bowl and mix until
smooth. Apply to clean, dry skin and let sit for 15–20
minutes. Rinse with warm water and pat dry.

DIY WINTER HAIR MASK

Deep Conditioning Aloe Hair Mask (for dry hair)

¼ cup avocado, mashed

¼ cup aloe vera gel

1–2 tablespoons olive oil
(you can sub with jojoba or
rosehip oil)

Mash avocado in a bowl and stir in the aloe vera gel and olive oil (or blend in a small blender). After shampooing, work the mask onto the ends of your hair. Leave mask in for 15–20 minutes (put on a shower cap if you have one), then rinse with warm water and condition if needed.

WINTER ESSENTIAL OIL BLENDS

2–3 drops each, or more as desired

GROUNDEDNESS: Cedarwood, Patchouli, and Sandalwood

FEMININE POWER: Bergamot and Geranium

DEEP RELAXATION: Lavender, Patchouli, Sweet Marjoram, Mandarin, Geranium, and Chamomile

INNER PEACE: Tangerine, Frankincense, and Sandalwood

NUTRITION

- During this phase, your body needs rich, comforting, and soothing foods to remineralize and replenish.

- Focus on foods that will keep your uterus warm like broths, stews or miso soups with tofu, kombu, and kelp.

- Restore your blood and kidneys with sea vegetables and foods rich in iron and zinc. Eat plenty of high-protein kidney beans, black beans, kale, kelp, nori, mushrooms, and beets.

- Add sea salt to your food and water to rebalance electrolytes and minerals.

- To help increase the absorption of iron, eat foods high in vitamin C such as dark berries, kale, broccoli, and bell peppers.

- To help eliminate excess water, focus on low-glycemic, water-rich fruits and veggies such as cucumber, watermelon, and grapes.

- Stir-fries with liquid aminos, tempeh, water chestnuts, mushrooms, and kale, or seaweed sushi rolls with nori, cucumber, brown rice, and tofu are great meal options.

- Choose dense, gluten-free grains such as buckwheat kasha, forbidden black rice, wild rice, or brown rice.

- Adding liquid chlorophyll to your water or smoothies will help to increase iron and help alleviate fatigue.

Winter Food Chart

VEGETABLES	GLUTEN-FREE GRAINS	NUTS AND SEEDS
beet	black rice	chestnut
dulse	brown rice	ground flaxseed
hijiki	buckwheat or kasha	hazelnut
kale	wild rice	pumpkin seed
kelp		
kombu		
mushrooms (any variety)		
nori		
wakame		
water chestnut		

FRUITS	LEGUMES	OTHER
blackberries	adzuki beans	bancha tea
blueberries	black beans	chlorella/liquid chlorophyll
cranberries	edamame* (organic)	coconut water
grapes	kidney beans	fennel tea
watermelon	natto	lemon water
	tempeh* (organic)	licorice tea
	tofu* (organic)	liquid aminos
		miso (organic)
	** Tempeh, tofu and eda-mame are soy products that must be purchased organic; otherwise, they are likely to be GMO.	sea salt
		tamari (low sodium)

WINTER RECIPES

Breakfast

HYDRATING DARK BERRY SMOOTHIE

(makes 1 serving)

2 handfuls of kale leaves

½ cup frozen blueberries or blackberries

½ cup frozen zucchini (chopped and steamed before freezing)

1 scoop vegan plain or vanilla plant protein

1 tablespoon chia seeds (can sub flax seeds)

1 ½ cups coconut water

Handful of ice (optional)

Add all ingredients to a high-speed blender. Blend until smooth.

GROUNDING SWEET BEET SMOOTHIE

(makes 1 serving)

Handful of kale leaves

½ of a fresh beet, peeled and cubed

½ of a frozen banana

1 scoop vegan plain or vanilla plant protein powder

1 tablespoon ground flaxseed

1 tablespoon almond butter

1 cup unsweetened vanilla almond milk + ½ cup water

Handful of ice (optional)

Add all ingredients to a high-speed blender. Blend until smooth.

BLACK BEAN TOFU SCRAMBLE

(makes 2 servings)

2 tablespoons avocado oil (can sub grapeseed or coconut oil)

1 shallot, finely diced

1 head of broccoli florets

1 cup chopped white button mushrooms (about 6)

1 clove minced garlic

1 14-ounce package organic extra-firm tofu

2 tablespoons nutritional yeast

1 teaspoon turmeric

2 teaspoons low-sodium tamari (or soy sauce/liquid aminos)

½ teaspoon sea salt (can sub kala namak or truffle salt)

½ teaspoon black pepper

½ teaspoon paprika

1 can black beans, drained and rinsed

2 cups chopped kale leaves

¼ cup chopped fresh cilantro

½ fresh lemon, squeezed

Optional toppings: dulse flakes, avocado, salsa

In a large pan, heat the avocado oil over medium-high heat. Once hot, sauté the shallot for about four minutes, or until translucent. Stir in the broccoli, mushrooms, and garlic, plus a pinch of salt and pepper. *Feel free to add in more veggies than the recipe calls for. I usually load up on veggies and use whatever I have on hand.* Turn heat down to medium and cover to steam the vegetables for about 4–5 minutes or until tender, but not overcooked. The broccoli should still be vibrant in color.

Meanwhile, crumble the tofu into a large bowl then mix in the spices, nutritional yeast, turmeric, tamari, sea salt, pepper, and paprika. Mix until well-combined, and the spices are evenly dispersed on the crumbled tofu. Stir the crumbled tofu into the pan with the veggies. Cook 5–10 minutes, then add in the black beans to warm for about two minutes. You will notice the golden color getting deeper. Add the kale, cilantro, and lemon, and remove from heat. Serve on gluten-free toast with avocado and/or salsa on the side, with rice or quinoa, or plain. Store leftovers in the refrigerator.

Note: no need to drain or remove excess water from tofu in this recipe as it creates more of a scramble-like texture.

SUNDAY MORNING GLUTEN-FREE BANANA PANCAKES

(makes 6–7 pancakes)

¾ cup gluten-free oat flour

½ cup buckwheat flour (it's gluten-free, can sub oat flour)

1 tablespoon ground flaxseed

2 teaspoons baking powder

2 teaspoons cinnamon

Pinch of sea salt

1 ¼ cup unsweetened vanilla almond milk (or any plant milk)

1 ripe banana, mashed (can sub for ½ cup unsweetened applesauce)

2 tablespoons melted coconut oil

2 tablespoon maple syrup (I use Choc Zero maple syrup)

½ tablespoon apple cider vinegar (or fresh lemon juice)

1 teaspoon vanilla extract (alcohol-free)

1 tablespoon coconut oil (for frying)

In a large bowl, whisk the oat flour, buckwheat flour, ground flaxseed, baking powder, cinnamon, and sea salt until well-combined. In a separate bowl, combine all of the wet ingredients—the almond milk, mashed banana, melted coconut oil, maple syrup, and vanilla. Whisk the wet ingredients together until smooth, then pour the wet ingredients into the dry mixture and stir until well-combined (add a couple tablespoons of water if too dry). Set mixture aside for 5 minutes to thicken.

Heat the coconut oil in a frying pan on the stove over medium heat. Once hot, pour ¼ cup of the pancake mixture onto the pan and cook until you see little bubbles popping, then gently flip to the other side and cook for 2–3 more minutes. Continue with the rest of the mixture.

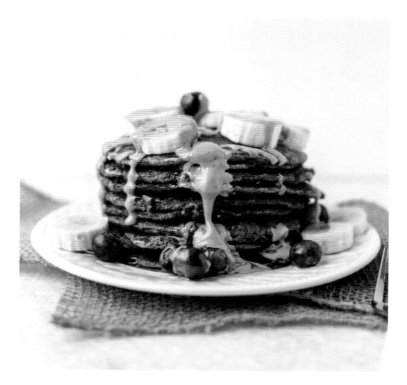

DECONSTRUCTED MERMAID SUSHI NORI BOWL (OR WRAP)

(makes 2 servings)

1 14-oz package organic extra-firm tofu

2-4 tablespoons low-sodium tamari (to marinate tofu) or liquid aminos

2 tablespoons rice vinegar, divided

½ cup uncooked short-grain brown rice (or 1 cup cooked)

½ cucumber, chopped

4 cups kale, chopped (can sub spinach)

1 tablespoon maple syrup

1 avocado, cubed

1–2 large nori seaweed sheets (or dulse flakes)

OPTIONAL TOPPINGS:
pickled ginger, green onion, sesame seeds, wasabi, dulse flakes

Begin by draining the package of tofu to remove excess water, then cut tofu lengthwise into four slices. Lay the slices flat over a couple of paper towels (or a clean kitchen towel) on top of a baking sheet. Lay a couple more paper towels over the tofu. Place another baking sheet (or heavy, flat-bottomed object) on top, plus a heavy book on top of that (because you don't want the book to get wet). Set aside for 20–30 minutes (note: you can also use a tofu press if you have one). After the tofu has been pressed, cube the tofu, transfer to a bowl and drizzle with tamari and 1 tablespoon of the rice vinegar. Set aside.

Prepare the brown rice by combining ½ cup brown rice with 1 cup water in a pot on the stove. Bring to a boil and cover, then reduce heat to simmer for 20 minutes, or until water is absorbed. After cooking, season the rice in the pot with a few splashes of liquid aminos and a roughly crumbled sheet of nori (or a handful of dulse flakes). Set aside.

You can cube the tofu and eat as-is or fry it in a pan with coconut oil. To fry, heat 2 teaspoons of coconut oil over medium-high heat. Once hot, add the cubed tofu and fry for five minutes on each side until lightly browned and crispy.

Before assembling the deconstructed sushi bowls, I like to soften the kale by adding the remaining 1 tablespoon rice vinegar with the maple syrup into a bowl and massaging it into the kale leaves. Then separate the kale into two bowls, and add the tofu, brown rice, and cucumber to each. Finish with avocado, extra crumbled nori, and a squeeze of lemon or lime.

Note: You can also roll all ingredients into a wrap with a large nori sheet. If you prefer to steam the kale instead of eating it raw, that is fine, too.

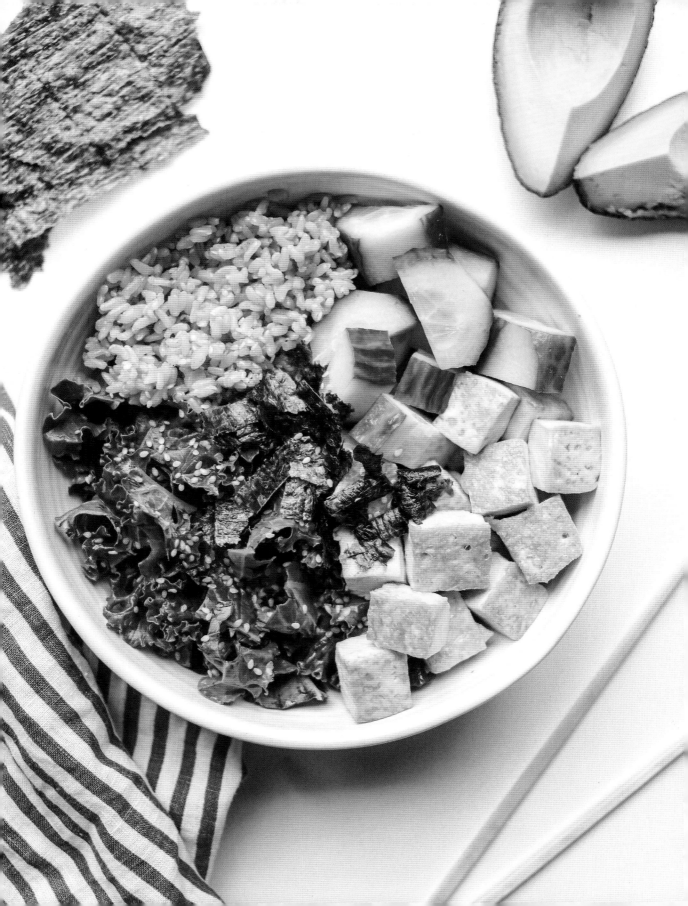

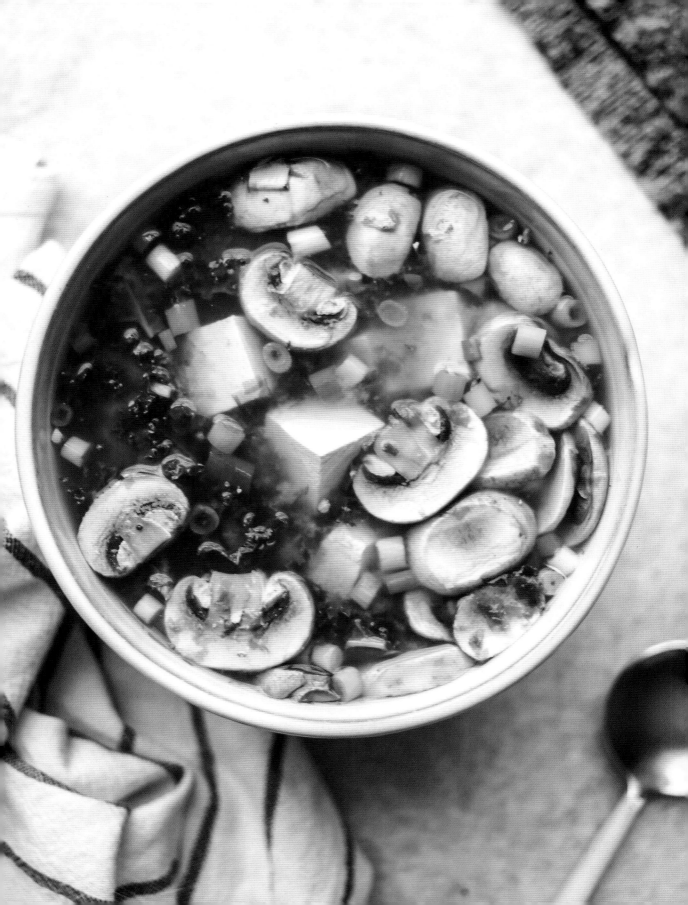

MOOD-LIFTING MISO SOUP

(makes 2 servings)

4 cups water

1 sheet nori, roughly crumbled or shredded

3 tablespoons white miso paste (fermented soybean paste)

1 cup chopped kale leaves, green Swiss chard or bok choy

1/2 cup chopped green onion

½ cup chopped mushrooms (any variety)

1 cup extra firm tofu (cubed) (½ block from a 14-ounce container)

Add water to a medium-sized pot and bring to a low simmer. Add the crumbled sheet of nori and simmer for 5 minutes. In the meantime, place miso into a small bowl, add 2–3 tablespoons of hot water (from the pot), and whisk until smooth to eliminate clumps. Set aside. Add kale (or whichever green you chose), green onion, mushrooms, and tofu to the pot and cook for five minutes. Remove from heat and stir in miso mixture. Taste and add more miso, a splash of tamari, or a pinch of sea salt, if desired. Serve.

Note: no need to drain or remove excess water from the tofu, as it is in soup and will absorb liquid anyway.

BBQ BLACK BEAN BURGERS

(makes 4 burgers)

1 cup cooked brown rice

2 tablespoons avocado oil, divided

½ medium white onion, finely chopped

1 cup raw walnuts

⅓ cup almond flour (or gluten-free bread crumbs)

3 tablespoons gluten-free oat flour

2 tablespoons ground flaxseed

1 tablespoon chili powder

1 tablespoon paprika

1 tablespoon cumin

½ teaspoon sea salt

½ teaspoon black pepper

1 tablespoon coconut sugar

1 15-oz can black beans, drained and rinsed

¼ cup of homemade Vegan BBQ Sauce (recipe on next page)

If brown rice is uncooked, prepare it by combining ½ cup brown rice with 1 cup water in a pot on the stove. Bring to a boil and cover, then reduce heat to simmer for 20 minutes, or until the water is absorbed.

Heat 1 tablespoon avocado oil in a large pan over medium heat. Once hot, stir in the onion. Season with a bit of salt and pepper and sauté for 3–4 minutes, or until onion is soft and translucent. Turn off heat and set aside.

Next, make the BBQ sauce by adding all of the BBQ sauce ingredients to a small bowl and whisking to combine until smooth. Set aside.

In a food processor, add walnuts and blend until it reaches a meal-like consistency. Then add in the almond flour, oat flour, ground flaxseed, chili powder, paprika, cumin, sea salt, pepper, and coconut sugar, and blend until well combined. Transfer to a large bowl and set aside. Add black beans to the food processor and pulse to mash them, leaving a few semi-whole beans for texture. Transfer beans to the large mixing bowl with the walnut mixture; add in the cooked brown rice, sautéed onion and ¼ cup of the BBQ sauce. Mix with a wooden spoon (or your hands) until a dough starts to form. If too dry, add 1–2 tablespoons water, and if too wet, add 1–2 tablespoons almond flour. Mold into 4 burgers.

Heat remaining 1 tablespoon of avocado oil in the same pan used earlier (for the onions) on medium heat. Once hot, add the burgers and cook for 3–4 minutes or until lightly browned. Gently flip over and cook another 3–4 minutes. Reduce heat if they are browning too quickly. Serve burgers on a gluten-free bun or in a collard wrap with extra BBQ sauce, and sweet potato fries or steamed veggies as a side.

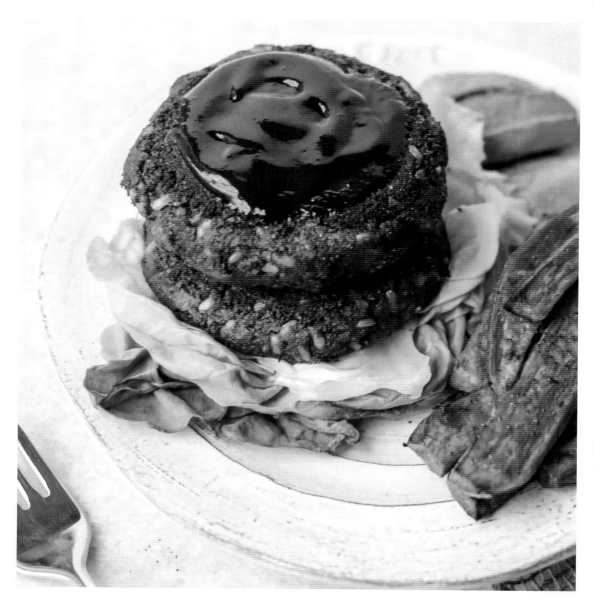

VEGAN BBQ SAUCE

(makes extra for topping)

1 cup organic ketchup

1 tablespoon molasses

2 tablespoons pure maple syrup

2 tablespoons apple cider vinegar

2 tablespoons low sodium tamari

1 tablespoon Sriracha, or other hot sauce

Combine all ingredients in a small bowl and mix until smooth.

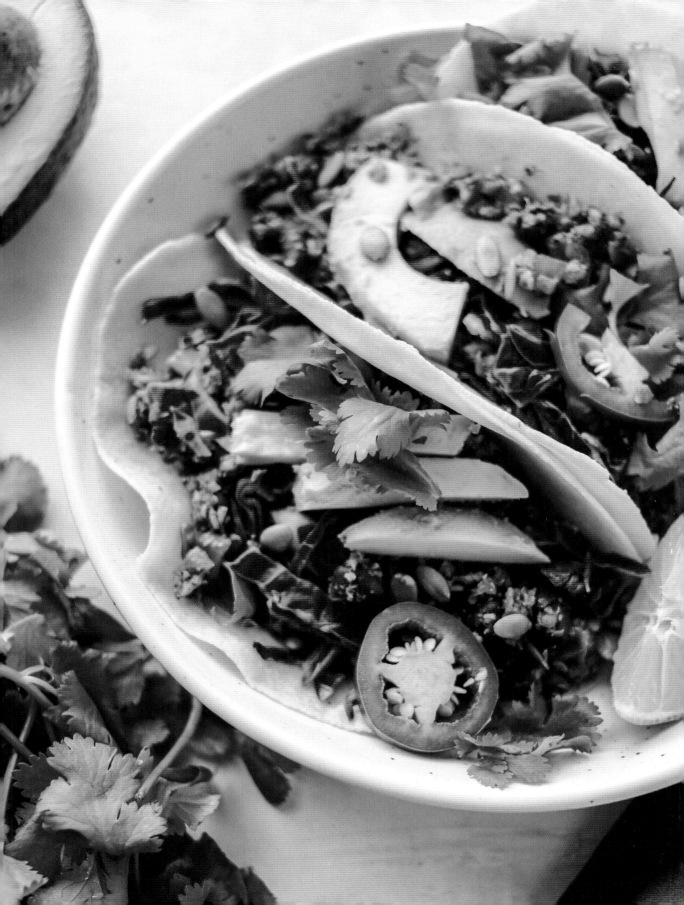

SPICY PORTOBELLO PEPITA TACOS

(makes 4 servings)

3 cups raw broccoli florets
(about 1 large head, or 2 small)

2 cups white button
mushrooms, washed and
stems removed (from one
8-ounce container)

1 ½ tablespoons coconut oil

½ white onion, finely diced

½ jalapeño, finely diced

2 cloves garlic, minced

1 cup raw pepitas
(pumpkin seeds)

2 teaspoons cumin

2 teaspoons chili powder

1 teaspoon cayenne (optional)

½ teaspoon sea salt

½ teaspoon black pepper

1 15-ounce can black beans,
drained and rinsed (can
substitute kidney beans)

½ cup fresh cilantro, chopped

Fresh juice of ½ lime (optional)

Corn tortillas (can substitute
whatever tortillas you prefer, or
use lettuce cups)

*Optional toppings: avocado,
tomato, cilantro, salsa, corn*

Use a food processor to blend the broccoli florets until they are crumbled, with no major chunks remaining. Add to a bowl. Do the same for the mushrooms and add to the same bowl. Set aside.

Heat the coconut oil in a pan on the stove over medium-high heat. Once hot, sauté the onion and jalapeño, about four minutes, then turn down heat to medium and stir in garlic, being careful not to burn. Then add the broccoli and mushrooms, and turn heat down to medium-low, occasionally stirring to soften and lightly sauté the veggies.

In the food processor, add the pepitas, cumin, chili powder, cayenne, salt, and pepper, and blend/pulse into a fine, meal-like consistency. Transfer mixture into the pan on the stove, along with the black beans. Turn the heat up to medium, cook for about 5–7 minutes, then turn off heat. Stir in cilantro and fresh lime.

Serve in corn tortillas with any toppings you desire or serve plain in a bowl alongside greens, with toppings.

SWEET FUDGY FLOURLESS FEEL-BETTER BROWNIES

(makes 8 brownies)

2 medium-sized ripe bananas, mashed

2 tablespoons runny almond butter (can sub any nut or seed butter)

2 tablespoons unsweetened applesauce (can sub for almond butter)

⅓ cup raw cacao powder

1 scoop vegan protein powder (chocolate or vanilla)

2 tablespoons vegan chocolate chips, plus more for topping

Preheat oven to 350 degrees. Whisk the mashed bananas, almond butter, and applesauce in a large bowl. Stir in the cacao powder and protein powder and mix until completely smooth. Stir in the chocolate chips.

Line a loaf pan with parchment paper or grease it with coconut oil and transfer the batter into the pan. It will be very thick—use a spatula to spread it out evenly. Sprinkle extra chocolate chips on top. Bake for 20–25 minutes. The brownies will seem underdone when you take them out, but they will firm up after cooling. Once cool, slice into eight squares.

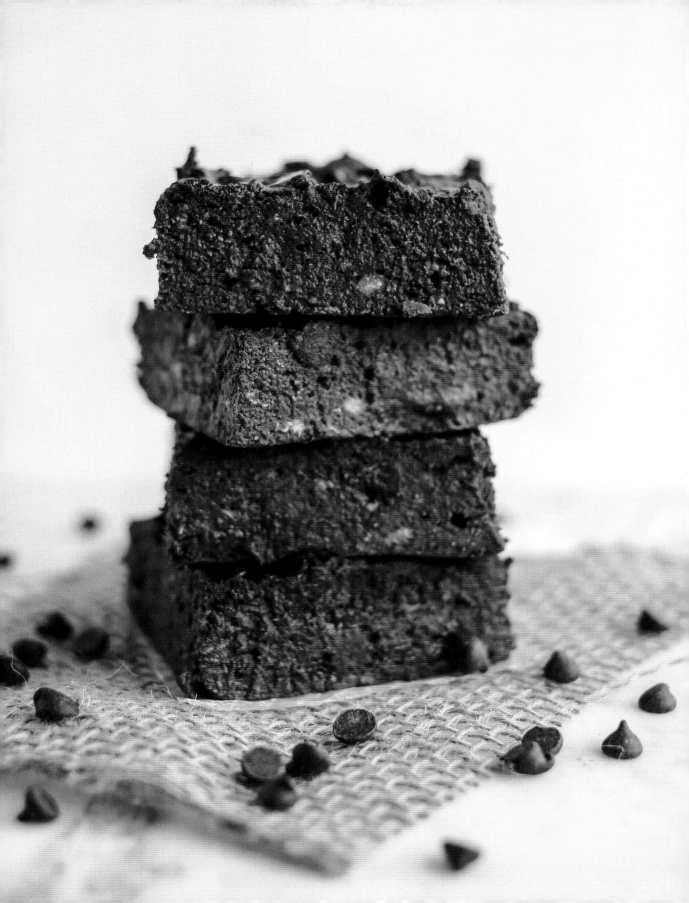

CHAPTER

10

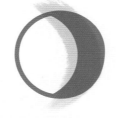

Phase Two:

FOLLICULAR

Spring | Waxing Moon

LASTS 7-10 DAYS
BBT: 97.0 - 97.7

SPRING IN YOUR BODY, AS IN NATURE, BRINGS a sense of growth, renewal, creation, and new beginnings. Your follicular phase is a fresh start, full of fresh air and light. This exciting phase helps prepare your body for ovulation. Since your period just ended, you're feeling optimistic, creative, and energized. You feel inclined to plan out your life and work for the next few weeks, leading up to your next period. During the follicular phase, your mood and brain function are optimized, which makes the planning process a breeze.

YOUR HORMONES

In the follicular phase, your body is preparing to release an egg during ovulation. Each ovary is filled with hundreds of thousands of follicles, and this phase is their final stage of development. A follicle is a sac of cells that contains an immature egg at the center. During the first seven days of your cycle, the pituitary gland is signaled to send FSH (follicle-stimulating hormone) to each ovary, which stimulates a number of follicles to grow (8–15 will grow in each ovary, on average). These maturing follicles release estradiol into the bloodstream to build up the endometrium (uterine lining) where the fertilized egg will implant, should fertilization occur. Estradiol is the best. Known as the "happy hormone," this female sex hormone increases the neurotransmitter serotonin, which boosts feelings of well-being and dopamine, boosting motivation. This leaves you feeling energized, confident, happy, and more outgoing.

After your period ends around day seven of your cycle, one follicle (or more rarely, two follicles) has won the great race and becomes the dominant follicle, while the other growing follicles start to degenerate. The dominant follicle continues to swell while nourishing the egg inside, in preparation to rupture and be released from the ovary for ovulation.

MOOD & ENERGY

To keep stress at bay throughout your cycle, it's imperative to take advantage of this time when planning feels effortless, fun, and productive. Your creative juices are flowing freely, and you feel ready to make decisions and take initiative. It's a great time to collaborate on new projects and be assertive with your ideas and goals. Try new things, problem solve, take bold risks, set new intentions, and brainstorm big plans. Tune into your vision for the future and gain clarity on the action steps you need to take to reach your goals.

Since you tend to learn things quicker in this phase, it's a great time to gain some new skills at work or take a class. Better yet, apply for that dream job you can't stop thinking about (be sure to schedule the interview near the Ovulation phase). Your actions don't all need to be work-related either—try a new art class, join a book club, take a cooking class—whatever sounds appealing to you. This is the time in your cycle when you tend to be future-focused and positive about what's ahead.

EXERCISE

This is the time to get active. Physically, the follicular phase is when you feel lightest, and the least weighed down. Keeping with the feelings of spring, renewal, and new beginnings, this is the best time to try a new workout, join a new gym, or mix things up with a group class you've been too nervous to try. Because your confidence is rising, you feel more open and less fearful, so take advantage of putting yourself out there in new fitness situations.

Energy is rising, so set out to challenge yourself. Focus on active, cardio-based workouts like dance classes, biking, hiking, rock climbing, swimming, rowing, boot camp, or fiery, fast-sequence yoga classes. *For at home workouts, I love the PopSugar Fitness YouTube channel during this phase for fun, upbeat workout videos.*

Checking Back in on New Habits

Starting something new during this phase means it will be more likely to stick and become a habit than in any other phase.

I want you to think back to this phase in 1-2 weeks during your luteal phase when you may feel unmotivated or have no desire to stick to a new goal. If you lose steam, don't be hard on yourself. It's not your fault. Only you know how far you can push yourself, and this may or may not be a time to force your willpower.

After reflecting, if you don't have the strength to keep going with a new plan, hobby or goal, it's okay. Things don't always stick, but at least you are trying new things and putting yourself out there. But don't force something that feels miserable. Women are way too hard on themselves, and I think that has far more health repercussions than honoring your body, brain chemistry, and where you are at a particular moment. You can always try again next month.

SEX

Coming off your period, hormones are at lower levels until estrogen starts to increase again a few days before ovulation. Because of this, you'll want to focus on stimulation and arousal to heighten your mood for sex. This is a great time to try something new in the bedroom, whether it be a new position, a new place, or whatever "new" means to you. Another great way to keep things fresh is to connect outside of the bedroom first and build intimacy by trying new activities like hiking, going to concerts, renting bikes to ride, or any new physical activity you can do together.

LUBRICATION

There will be little to no cervical mucus for the first few days after your period ends. You'll feel dry until estrogen starts to rise which can happen anywhere from day 6 to day 12, and it's different for each woman. It is then that you may notice a pattern of discharge that develops more fertile characteristics leading up to ovulation. Starting out, it may feel sticky, flaky, and somewhat springy, but it won't feel wet. Then, it will change to a wetter type that looks white and creamy. This type of discharge is considered the transitional type that leads to fertile mucus in the next phase. Until then, it is still considered a dry phase, meaning the types of discharge are not ideal lubrication for sex. You may consider supplementing with lubricant.

SKIN

This phase (and the ovulation phase) is your skin's time to shine. New skin cells are forming, and your skin feels fresh with improved elasticity. Now is an excellent time to get facials, extractions, or do any skin treatment. Your skin is less prone to redness and won't feel as sensitive thanks to increasing estrogen, so it's also the best time for a bikini wax.

DIY SPRING FACE MASK

Probiotic Lemon Brightening Turmeric Mask

2 tablespoons plain
coconut yogurt

1 tablespoon oat flour (can sub
rolled oats)

½ teaspoon ground turmeric

squeeze of lemon

Combine all ingredients in a small bowl and mix until well-combined. Apply to clean, dry skin and let sit for 15 minutes. Rinse with warm water and pat dry.

Note: your skin may look like it's stained yellow but no need to worry! If it does, wash again with a gentle cleanser and rinse.

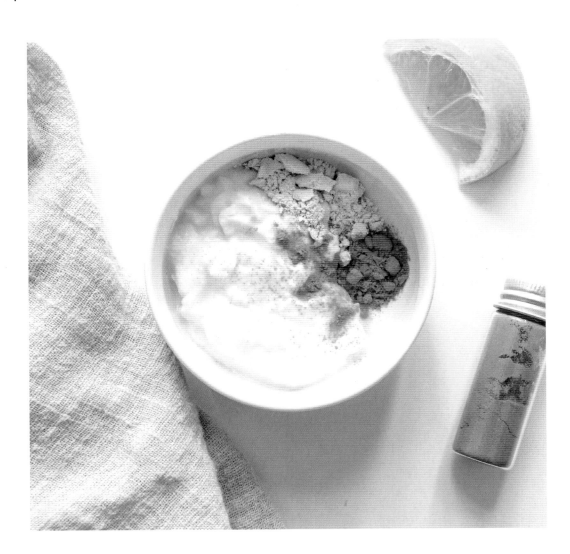

DIY SPRING HAIR MASK

Smooth Shine Apple Cider Vinegar Hair Rinse (restores pH balance)

¼ cup apple cider vinegar

2 tablespoons filtered water

1 tablespoon lemon juice

Pour hair rinse over cleansed, wet hair and work into scalp. Leave on for 10 minutes. Rinse with warm water. There is no need to condition afterward.

SPRING ESSENTIAL OIL BLENDS

2–3 drops each, or more as desired

ENERGIZING: Grapefruit, Lemon, Peppermint

SPRING BREAK: Sandalwood and Lime (also smells like key lime pie)

EARLY RISER: Grapefruit and Basil

NEW BEGINNINGS: Lemongrass, Eucalyptus, Rosemary

NUTRITION

As estrogen starts to rise, it may contribute to a lack of appetite. This is normal, which is why eating higher fat and colorful fresh foods to feed your follicles feels good at this time. Think extra avocado and vibrant vegetables like carrots, broccoli, zucchini, or green beans.

- ☐ Eat more vitamin-C rich citrus fruits like grapefruit, oranges, nectarines, lemons or limes (all the lemon water), as well as cherries, plums, and pomegranates.

- ☐ Increase your healthy fat intake with avocados, olives, and nut butter to add to your increasing energy.

- ☐ Add vinegar (like raw apple cider vinegar or raw coconut vinegar) to your meals or use vinegar-based dressings and sauces.

- ☐ Probiotic-rich foods will prime your digestion for the month. Think pickled veggies, raw sauerkraut, kimchi, and dairy-free, unsweetened yogurt (in the form of coconut, almond, or cashew).

- ☐ Also, eat a lot of greens with light lettuces like Romaine, Bibb, or Boston. For a more energizing salad, add lightly steamed or sautéed vegetables, sprouted lentils, or a sprouted grain (sprouted varieties are easier to digest, due to their activated enzymes).

- ☐ Make oatmeal with gluten-free oats, ground flaxseed, goji berries, and cashew butter.

- ☐ Choose sourdough bread, sprouted rye toast, or any sprouted bread and spread avocado on top.

Spring Food Chart

VEGETABLES	GRAINS	NUTS AND SEEDS
artichokes asparagus basil broccoli carrots green beans green peas lettuce (Romaine, Bibb, Boston) parsley snow peas sprouts (alfalfa, kale, broccoli, etc.) sugar snap peas zucchini	amaranth barley (contains gluten) farro (contains gluten) oats (look for a gluten-free variety) teff quinoa	brazil nuts cashews (cashew butter) flaxseeds (ground) macadamia nuts pumpkin/pepita seeds

FRUITS	LEGUMES	OTHER
avocados grapefruit cherries clementines lemons limes lychees mandarins (not canned) nectarines oranges plums pomegranates	black-eyed peas edamame* lentils (any variety) lima beans mung beans split pea tempeh* tofu* *Tempeh, tofu, and edamame are soy products that must be purchased organic; otherwise, they are likely GMO products.*	dairy-free yogurt unsweetened (coconut, almond or cashew) goji berries nut butter (cashew or your favorite kind, for extra fat during this phase!) capers olives pickles pickled veggies raw sauerkraut vinegar (apple cider, balsamic, champagne, coconut, red wine, etc.)

SPRING RECIPES

Breakfast

ENERGIZING SPRING BREAK SHAKE

(makes 1 serving)

2 large handfuls spinach

¼ avocado (or 2 tablespoons
raw cashews)

1-inch chunk fresh ginger (or 1
tablespoon dried ginger)

1 scoop vegan unflavored or
vanilla protein powder

1 tablespoon ground flaxseed

Fresh juice of ½ lemon (or lime)

½ tablespoon raw apple
cider vinegar

1 ½ cups plain coconut water or
filtered water

Handful of ice (optional)

OPTIONAL TOPPINGS:
broccoli sprouts and/or
extra lemon

Add all ingredients to a high–speed blender. Blend
until smooth.

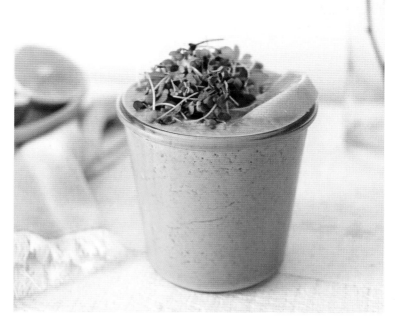

COCONUT CASHEW SMOOTHIE

(makes 1 serving)

½ frozen banana

½ cup chopped frozen zucchini, optional (steamed then frozen for easier digestion)

1 scoop vegan plant protein powder (vanilla or plain)

1 tablespoon ground flaxseed

½ teaspoon ground cinnamon

2 tablespoons shredded coconut (unsweetened)

2 tablespoons raw cashews (or 2 tablespoons cashew butter)

1 cup unsweetened vanilla almond milk

½ cup filtered water (omit if you want a thicker consistency)

OPTIONAL SMOOTHIE TOPPINGS: a drizzle of cashew butter, shredded coconut, granola or crushed cashews, for crunch

Add all ingredients to a high–speed blender. Blend until smooth.

BRAZIL NUT PROBIOTIC YOGURT BOWL

(makes 1 serving)

1 cup plain coconut yogurt (or any plain, unsweetened dairy-free yogurt with minimal ingredients)

1 tablespoon ground flaxseed or chia seeds

Splash of unsweetened almond, coconut or cashew milk

5-6 drops of stevia (optional)

3-4 crushed brazil nuts (or pepitas)

¼ cup pomegranate seeds (or ½ cup cherries or ½ of a peeled grapefruit)

Assemble your yogurt bowl by mixing yogurt with flaxseed or chia seeds, a splash of almond milk and stevia; top with crushed brazil nuts and your choice of fruit.

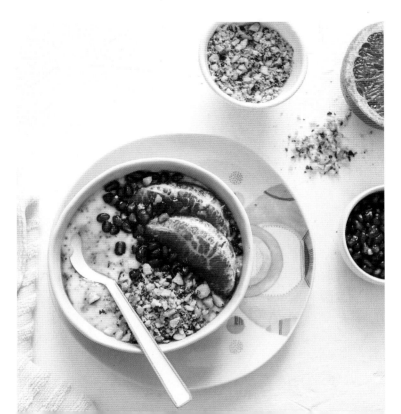

CREAMY CHOCOCADO PUDDING

(makes 2 servings)

1 large ripe avocado

1 ripe medium-sized banana

⅓ cup raw cacao powder

⅓ cup cashew butter (or any nut butter)

2 tablespoons maple syrup (can sub coconut sugar or monk fruit granulated sweetener)

Pinch of sea salt

½ cup unsweetened vanilla almond milk or cashew milk (plus 2-3 tablespoons water if too thick)

OPTIONAL TOPPINGS:
a spoonful of coconut cream, crushed brazil nuts, or pepitas, a drizzle of cashew butter

Combine all ingredients in a food processor and blend until smooth and creamy. Serve in a bowl and store the other serving in the fridge for tomorrow's breakfast.

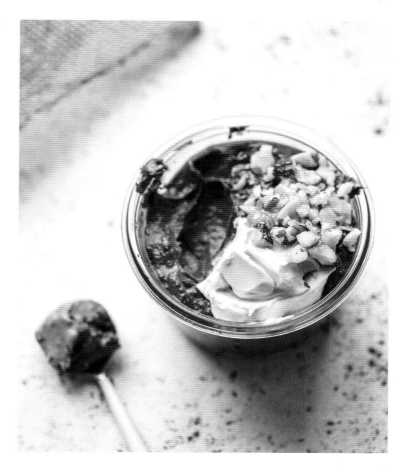

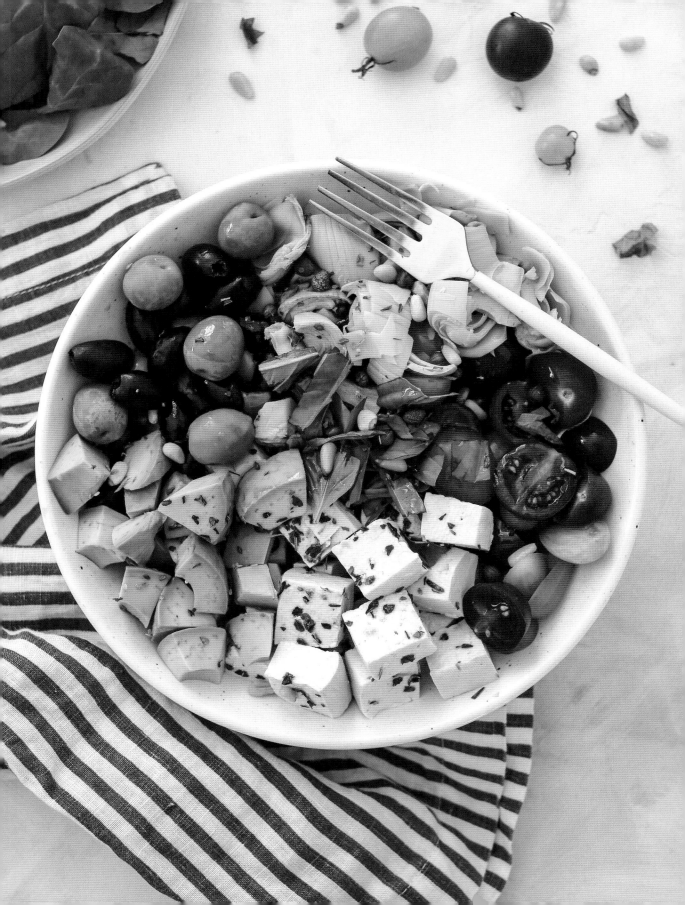

TOFU AVOCADO CAPRESE SALAD

(makes 2-3 servings)

1 block organic extra-firm tofu, drained and cubed into bite-size pieces

½ lemon, juiced

2 tablespoons extra-virgin olive oil

2 teaspoons dried Italian herb seasoning

2 cups grape tomatoes, halved (or one pint of tomatoes)

½ cup pitted olives, halved (I used a mix of Kalamata and Castelvetrano olives)

1 14-oz can of artichokes, drained and chopped

¼ cup chopped fresh basil

½ avocado, cubed

Begin by draining the package of tofu to remove excess water, then cut tofu lengthwise into four slices. Lay the slices flat over a couple of paper towels (or a clean kitchen towel) on top of a baking sheet. Lay a couple more paper towels over the tofu. Place another baking sheet (or a heavy flat-bottomed object) on top, plus a heavy book on top of that (because you don't want the book to get wet). Set aside for 20-30 minutes (note: you can also use a tofu press if you have one). Then, marinate tofu in lemon, olive oil, and Italian herb seasoning for 5 minutes. Meanwhile, prepare the rest of the salad by assembling the remaining ingredients in a bowl—the tomatoes, olives, artichokes, fresh basil, and avocado. Add in the tofu after it marinates. Serve over greens (like spinach) or quinoa. Refrigerate leftovers.

SPRING LENTIL LETTUCE CUPS WITH VEGAN HEMP RANCH

(makes 2 servings)

1 cup uncooked green lentils

2 cups filtered water

1 tablespoon coconut oil or avocado oil

⅓ white onion, chopped

½ jalapeño, optional

1 cup zucchini (finely diced)

1 tablespoon paprika

½ teaspoon sea salt

½ tablespoon raw apple cider vinegar

1 ripe mango, cubed

1 cup shredded carrots

Butter lettuce

OPTIONAL TOPPINGS:
Vegan Hemp Ranch (recipe on next page), sliced avocado, pepitas, broccoli sprouts, raw sauerkraut

I love serving these lettuce cups with guava kombucha, as pictured.

In a medium-sized pot, combine lentils with water and bring to a boil, then reduce heat to simmer for 15-20 minutes, or until water is absorbed and lentils are soft. In a separate small saucepan, heat oil on medium-high heat and sauté the onion, occasionally stirring for 3-4 minutes. Add the jalapeño, zucchini, paprika, and sea salt and cook for 8-9 minutes, or until zucchini softens. Turn off heat and stir in apple cider vinegar. Assemble each lettuce cup with lentils, mango, shredded carrot, avocado, and optional *Vegan Hemp Ranch* (see next page).

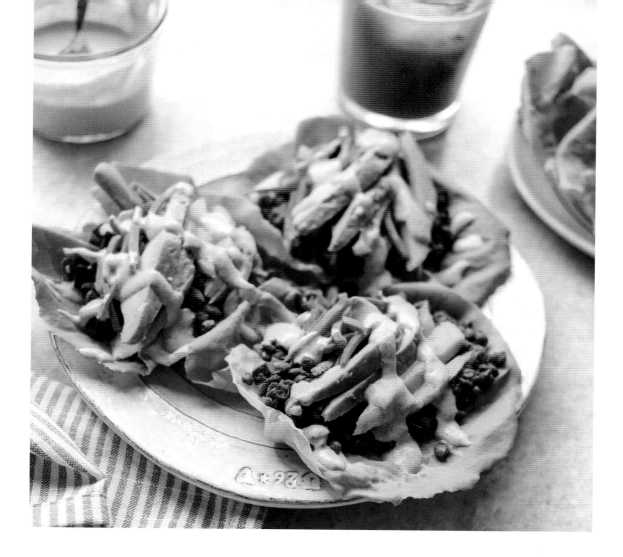

VEGAN HEMP RANCH

(makes 3-4 servings)

⅓ cup hemp hearts

⅓ cup raw cashews

2 tablespoons extra virgin olive oil

1 ½ tablespoons raw apple cider vinegar

1 clove garlic

1 teaspoon sea salt

1 teaspoon dried dill (or 1 tablespoon fresh dill)

1 handful fresh parsley

1 tablespoon chopped green onion

½ cup filtered water

In a small blender or a food processor, combine all ingredients and blend until smooth and creamy. If too thick, add 1–2 tablespoons water until you reach desired consistency.

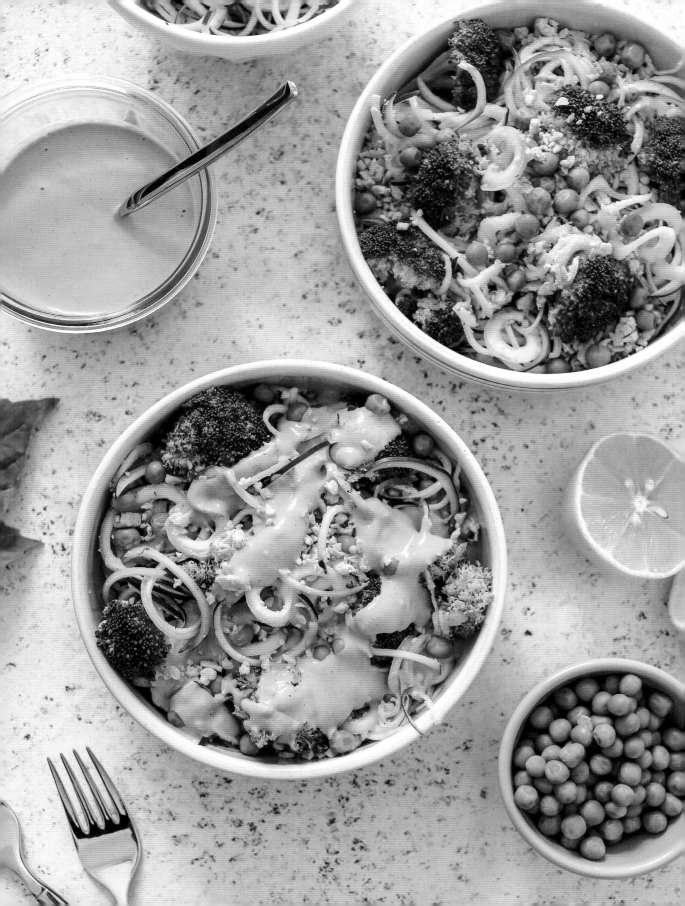

ZOODLE BROCCOLI BOWL WITH LEMON BASIL PESTO SAUCE

(makes 2 servings)

1 large zucchini (or 2 small)

⅔ package tempeh, crumbled

2 cups broccoli florets (from about 1 large head of broccoli)

1 cup frozen green peas (optional)

LEMON BASIL PESTO SAUCE

1 ½ cup fresh basil

1 ½ fresh lemons, juiced

Handful of spinach (optional)

3 tablespoons nutritional yeast

2 tablespoons pine nuts

2 tablespoons cashews

2 teaspoons red pepper flakes (or ½ jalapeño)

2 tablespoons avocado oil (or extra virgin olive oil)

½ teaspoon sea salt + ½ teaspoon black pepper

2 tablespoons water

Using a spiralizer, spiralize zucchini to make zucchini noodles. Set aside. Remove tempeh from the package and crumble into bite-sized pieces into a bowl. Set aside.

Add 1–2 inches of water to a medium-sized pot. Add steamer basket and place broccoli and peas in the basket. Bring water to a boil and cover to steam for about five minutes, or until veggies are soft. Meanwhile, make the Lemon Basil Pesto Sauce by combining all ingredients in a small blender or a food processor and blending until smooth and creamy. Assemble your bowl with zoodles, tempeh, steamed broccoli, and peas, then drizzle the pesto sauce on top.

SWEET AND SOUR MACRO BOWL

(makes 2-3 servings)

1 package tempeh, cubed (can also use 1 ½ cups shelled edamame)

1 bunch asparagus, chopped (can substitute green beans)

½ cup shredded carrots, per bowl

2 cups spinach, per bowl

Optional toppings: Pickled ginger, raw sauerkraut, crushed cashews, chopped green onion

Note: you can also add ½ cup cooked quinoa to make this recipe more filling.

SWEET AND SOUR SAUCE

3 tablespoons ketchup (or tomato paste)

1–2 tablespoons coconut sugar, to desired sweetness (or pure maple syrup)

1–2 tablespoons Sriracha

1 tablespoon rice vinegar (or apple cider vinegar)

1 tablespoon low-sodium gluten-free tamari (or liquid aminos)

2 teaspoons tapioca starch (arrowroot or cornstarch)

¼ cup + 2 tablespoons filtered water

Remove tempeh from package and cube into bite-sized pieces. Set aside. Combine all ingredients for Sweet and Sour Sauce in a small bowl and whisk until smooth. Transfer to a small pot and heat on medium-low heat to thicken, whisking occasionally. Once thickened (after about 10–15 minutes), stir in the tempeh until all pieces are coated, to warm. Wash and chop asparagus. Add 1–2 inches of water to a medium-sized pot and place steamer basket in a pot (or omit if you don't have one) and place asparagus and shredded carrots in the basket. Bring water to a boil then cover to steam for about five minutes, or until asparagus and carrots are soft.

Assemble your bowl with spinach, steamed veggies, sweet and sour tempeh, and any toppings you desire.

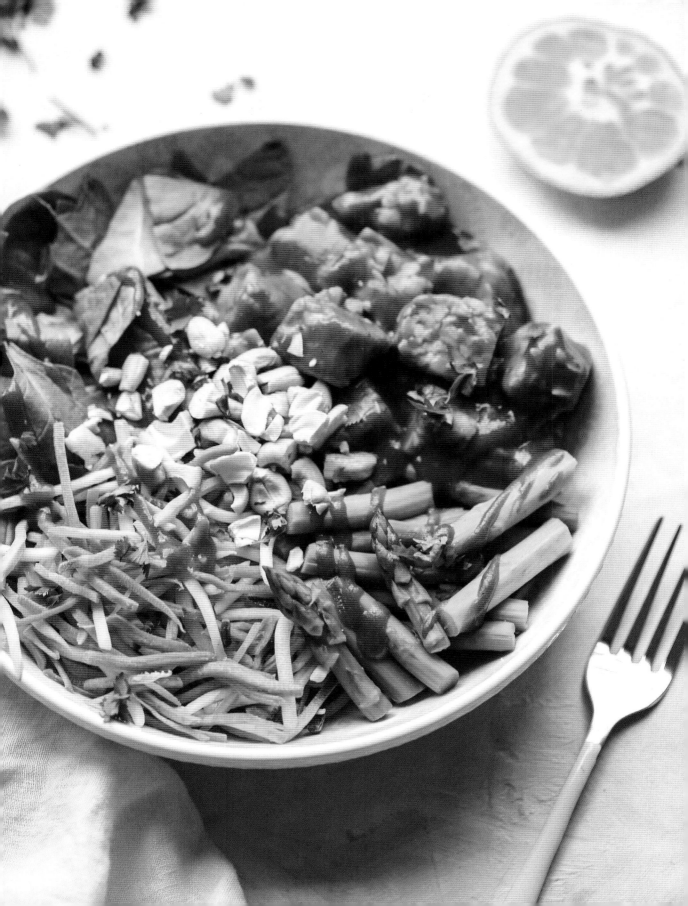

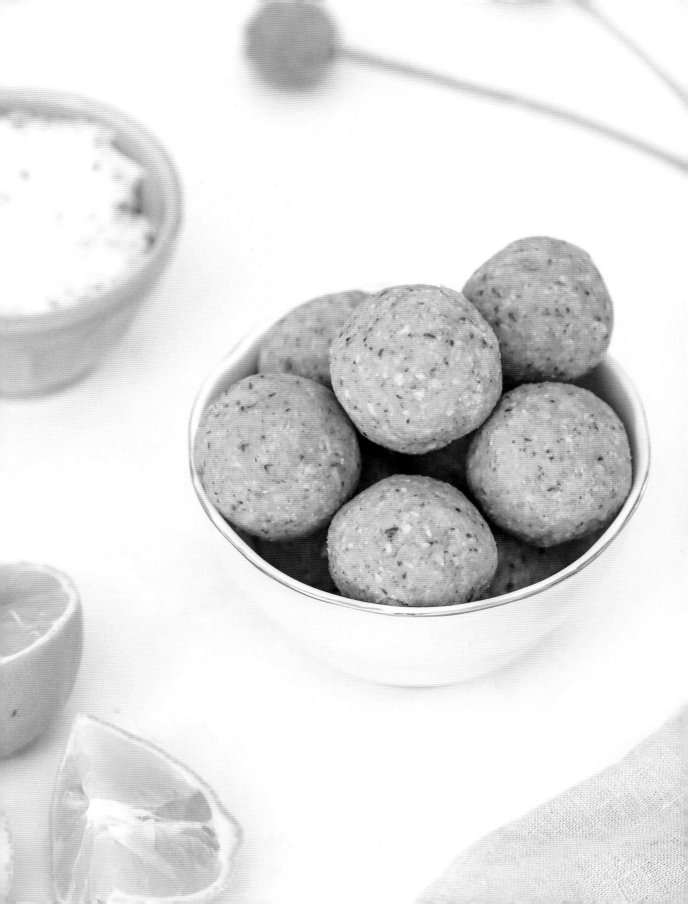

LEMON COOKIE BLISS BITES

(makes 12 balls)

1 cup raw cashews

¾ cup shredded coconut (unsweetened)

Pinch of sea salt

3 tablespoons coconut flour

½ tablespoon ground flaxseed

¼ teaspoon ground turmeric

¼ cup fresh lemon juice + optional 1 tablespoon lemon zest

2 tablespoons maple syrup

1 tablespoon melted coconut oil

½ teaspoon vanilla extract (alcohol-free)

In a food processor, add the cashews and coconut and blend until finely ground. Add the rest of the ingredients and pulse until the mixture is well combined and clumps into one big ball in the food processor bowl. Gently press into balls (they are too delicate to roll) and refrigerate for a couple of hours to harden.

CHAPTER

11

Phase Three:

OVULATORY

Summer | Full Moon

LASTS 3-4 DAYS
BBT: 97.0 - 97.7

SUMMERTIME IS ALL ABOUT BEING PLAYFUL AND HAVING FUN, and your body feels the same. The ovulation phase influences you to connect and be more social, which works perfectly as this is the peak of your cycle. This is when you are a magnet for desire and attention. It is also when you are most fertile, which is something to keep in mind. Think of this as the fun and flirty phase when you feel more outgoing, sexy, and beautiful than any other phase (if only it lasted all month).

Your skin is glowing, plump, and generally clear. The whites of your eyes look brighter, you probably have good hair days, and life feels effortless. Also, you'll have all the energy for intense workouts in the gym or in bed. Yes, this phase is also when you are most often in the mood. Plus, your partner desires you back because they're drawn to you on a biological level. Nature knows. Studies show that you are perceived as more attractive and desirable during this phase. Your five senses may also become more heightened.

YOUR HORMONES

Things are heating up. Around day 12, the dominant follicle secretes a surge of estrogen into the bloodstream, which prompts the hypothalamus to signal the pituitary gland to flood the bloodstream with luteinizing hormone (LH). Testosterone also peaks around this time, to spark sexual arousal. Around day 14, LH causes the dominant follicle to grow rapidly, and right before ovulation, the egg detaches from the dominant follicle which finally ruptures, releasing the egg. This is called ovulation, and the whole process is fairly quick and robust. You may feel a sudden twinge or sharp pain on one or both sides of your lower abdomen, depending on which ovary the egg is released from. Then, the egg is quickly and gently swept up by the fimbria of the fallopian tube and guided to the uterus by muscular contractions from the walls of the fallopian tube. The egg lives for 12-24 hours, which is the window when fertilization can occur. If not fertilized, the egg will disintegrate and shed with the uterine lining during bleeding.

Ovulation either happens, or it doesn't—there is no in between. It is a vital sign of general health and vitality. It means the body has been properly nourished, your stress is regulated, insulin levels are normal, and you have a well-functioning thyroid. Ovulation is the only way our bodies can produce progesterone, which is secreted from the corpus luteum. The endocrine gland is formed from the emptied follicle from which the egg was released. Progesterone is necessary for healthy bones, brain function, optimal metabolism, mood stabilization, and more (see Luteal Phase chapter).

MOOD & ENERGY

This is the phase when you have the most natural energy and are a magnet for desire. It's the best time to go out, be social and make connections. This is a time when you're self-assured, assertive, and your mood is stable. Words also come easily, so take advantage of your fierce communication skills and schedule presentations during this phase, go on that interview for your dream job, go on a first date, or attend networking events. If you've been putting off a hard conversation, now is a good time to have it since you are better able to get your message and opinion across without stumbling over your words. You are also more approachable, friendly, open-minded and sympathetic, which is essential for good, productive communication.

Because high levels of estrogen drive your desire for connection, you may feel inclined to say yes to social invitations and networking events, which is great—just be sure to check the calendar and see which phase you'll be in during the event. If it's during your follicular or ovulatory phase, then great. If not, you may want to reconsider how you respond. We can't say no to everything just because we're not in the most optimal phase for social events but honoring where your body will be later in the month is important (and you'll thank yourself later). I've made this mistake one too many times, where I respond *yes* to an event, only to dread it when the time comes. These are important aspects to consider when scheduling because we *do not* feel the same every week.

EXERCISE

Now is the time to go all out with high-impact workouts, take advantage of that soaring, natural energy. Think HIIT (high-intensity interval training) workouts, cardio, spin classes, running, circuit training, kickboxing, hot yoga, heavy weight lifting, plyometrics, boot camp classes—or sex. Engage in any sweaty, intense workouts to burn off that high energy. Group classes are great options too, since connecting and socializing with others feels natural. Push yourself. *For at-home extra-sweaty videos, I love the Fitness Blender YouTube channel, especially for HIIT workouts.*

SEX

You feel sexy, your libido is high, and your hormones are soaring. You're definitely in the mood during this phase, so think passionate, playful, and spicy in the bedroom. Because your chance of conceiving is at its highest, be sure to use a barrier method or protection to prevent pregnancy (see non-hormonal birth control, page 56), or abstain from intercourse altogether throughout this time.

Fertile mucus is at its peak in the days leading up to ovulation (consider fertile mucus a healthy pre-ovulation sign), which makes having sex more enjoyable. But keep in mind, it's meant to enhance fertility as it helps keep sperm inside you for up to five days. This is why you must practice caution during this phase if you're trying to avoid pregnancy (even if you have unprotected sex 3–4 days *before* ovulation, there's a chance of becoming pregnant due to the stretchy cervical fluid that protects and nourishes sperm while they await ovulation). On the other hand, if you are trying to conceive, now is the best time to get busy because fertile mucus also assists sperm in their journey to your egg.

LUBRICATION

In the 2–3 days leading up to ovulation, you'll notice fertile mucus because it can leave a circle of wet fluid on your underwear due to its high water content. Fertile mucus is slippery, stringy, and very stretchy, similar to the look and feel of raw egg whites. You may also notice it on toilet paper after you wipe. Ovulation is considered a wet phase, meaning this type of fluid (fertile mucus) is ideal lubrication for sex.

If you see fertile mucus *after* ovulation, which usually happens on days 14–17 of a 28-day cycle, it may mean you are not making enough progesterone to dry up the fluid. This may be your clue to do a hormone panel and test hormone levels (see page 32).

Note: A hormone-based IUD (or any progestin-type birth control) will inhibit the creation of fertile mucus. Read more about hormonal birth control in chapter 3.

The Physical Signs of Ovulation

Fertile mucus and regular periods are healthy signs of ovulation, although not concrete. An *anovulatory* cycle is possible, which means a cycle with a menstrual period but without ovulation. The average day for ovulation is 14, but this can vary if you have a longer cycle. To determine your possible date of ovulation, count back two weeks from the first heavy day of your period (another reason it's important to track your cycle).

A definite sign that ovulation occurred is a rise in waking BBT (see page 57) for three consecutive days *after* ovulation. So yes, you can only detect ovulation after the fact. Pre-ovulation, your waking temperature should be anywhere between 97.0 - 97.7 degrees. Post-ovulation, your waking temperature will rise by about 0.5 degrees and will hover there until your period. This may seem like a minimal temperature increase, but it's a significant sign that you did ovulate. This rise in temperature also lets you know you cannot become pregnant for the rest of this cycle, which is a pretty handy tool.

Another hint that ovulation may occur is a spike in sex drive in the days leading up to the egg release, due to a testosterone spike.

As mentioned earlier, another sign associated with ovulation is a sharp pain or cramping on one side or across your lower abdomen. This is also known as *mittelschmerz* and comes from the German words for "middle" and "pain" (because the sharp pain is felt during the middle of your cycle when an egg ruptures from a follicle in one of your ovaries). Some women don't feel a thing, while others recognize this sharp burst as a tell-tale sign that they're ovulating. Ovulation may alternate sides each month or favor one side for several months in a row. Some months you may feel it, others you may not. Because the pain is short-lived and coming from a natural process in your body, it's not something to be concerned about (unless of course, the pain is so severe, then you may be dealing with endometriosis or PCOS). While it is not entirely clear what causes the pain, it may be associated with either the swelling of one dominant follicle, the rupture of the ovarian wall to release the egg, muscle contractions surrounding the ovary, or muscle contractions of the fallopian tube to guide the egg toward the uterus.

ANOVULATION (LACK OF OVULATION)

Lack of ovulation is a cause of infertility, but also a reason for many common period symptoms and hormonal conditions. An anovulatory cycle may happen once in a while due to high stress levels, transitions, illnesses, coming off the birth control pill or medication, or even airplane travel, but it shouldn't be an ongoing occurrence. Your body knows when it's not an ideal time to reproduce, but because ovulation is the only way your body makes progesterone it's important to ovulate regularly for a healthy cycle. Hormonal birth control disrupts this process, so if you are on the pill, you are not ovulating and missing out on the health benefits of progesterone from natural ovulation.

Anovulation can be complicated and should involve a comprehensive, whole-body healing approach. I could write a second book on it. It can be caused by chronic stress, adrenal fatigue, underlying chronic inflammation, insulin resistance, food sensitivities (gluten or dairy), or thyroid disease. Lastly, anovulation may stem from a lack of proper nourishment due to not eating enough calories or food (specifically, carbs), not eating enough variety (which can lead to nutrient deficiencies), or having body fat that is too low (the ideal range for women is 18-24%). If you suspect you aren't ovulating, it's better to address the possible reasons why, especially if you plan on having a family.

To promote ovulation, make sure your diet is full of plenty of nutrient-dense, ovulation-promoting foods such as avocados (lots of them—like one per day), leafy greens, sprouted sunflower seeds, flaxseed, buckwheat, and chickpeas, as well as anti-inflammatory spices such as cinnamon and turmeric. Limiting caffeine and alcohol and quitting sugar are some of the best ways to support your body's natural rhythm to promote ovulation. You can mention this to your doctor if you suspect you aren't ovulating, but if you want help getting to the root issue of why you aren't ovulating, it is best to meet with a functional medicine doctor or naturopath. *See the Boost Fertility supplement section on page 91.*

HEALTH BENEFITS OF OVULATION

Even if you aren't trying for a baby right now, ovulation is good for you. Here are a few reasons why:

- ☐ Estrogen prevents bone loss and progesterone stimulates bone growth. It's the interplay of these two hormones that leads to optimal bone health for women, so they are prepared for menopause later in life. Without regular ovulation, the strength and health of your bones are compromised, which can lead to osteoporosis down the road.

- ☐ Progesterone plays a role in preventing breast cancer. Studies show that while estrogen stimulates breast cell growth, progesterone stimulates these cells to differentiate, allowing for maturation of cells for milk production. This means that without ovulation and without progesterone to keep them in line, breast cells may grow erratically and possibly lead to an overgrowth of abnormal or cancerous cells, posing a risk for breast cancer.

- ☐ Regular ovulation through your reproductive years can reduce the risk of heart disease later in life. A large study compared women with heart disease to those without heart disease. More of those with heart disease had low levels of progesterone, similar to anovulatory levels, than those without heart disease. This suggests that older women with heart disease are more likely to have had lower progesterone and thus more anovulatory cycles earlier in life. Evidence shows that progesterone is beneficial for heart disease risk factors, and some clinical studies suggest that regular ovulation prevents heart attacks later in life.

SKIN

The 2–3 days leading up to ovulation tend to be your best skin days. Pores minimize, skin is radiant, and the texture is refined. If you like the fresh-faced look, this is the time to embrace your skin *au naturale* or stick with lighter makeup. Let your gorgeous skin shine through. Your highest rates of estrogen contribute to that natural glow. Moisture levels are high, and there's an increase in collagen, so skin feels plump and youthful. If you're feeling too oily, be sure to exfoliate. And always remove makeup every night to prevent breakouts.

If you *are* experiencing breakouts during this time, excess estrogen could be the cause. Get a good sweat sesh in at the gym, dry brush to keep the lymphatic system moving (see page 45), and follow my food recommendations for each phase. Also, a great way to flush excess estrogen is some pleasure time alone or with a partner (perfect for your high libido in this phase), as regular orgasms help drain your lymphatic system. (See more about estrogen detoxification in the luteal phase chapter, page 199).

DIY SUMMER FACE MASK

Pink Strawberry Glow Mask

1 mashed strawberry

1 tablespoon coconut yogurt

1 tablespoon almond meal

½ tablespoon maple syrup

Combine all ingredients in a small bowl and mix until well-combined. Apply to clean, dry skin and let sit for 15 minutes. Rinse with warm water and pat dry.

DIY SUMMER HAIR MASK

Coconut Milk Reparative Moisture Hair Mask

1 banana, mashed

⅓ cup coconut milk

1 tablespoon olive oil (apply to ends of hair)

Mash banana in a small bowl and mix in coconut milk (or blend in small blender). Add olive oil to a separate small bowl. Work the fruit mixture into cleansed, wet hair, massaging it into hair for 4–5 minutes. Then work the olive oil into the ends of the hair only. Rinse thoroughly.

SUMMER ESSENTIAL OIL BLENDS

2–3 drops each, or more as desired

SWEET SUMMER: Sweet Orange and Ylang Ylang

ROMANCE: Lemon and Jasmine

ESSENCE OF SUMMER: Tangerine and Lemongrass

APHRODISIAC: Ylang Ylang, Patchouli, Sweet Orange, Lavender, Jasmine, Sandalwood

NUTRITION

Food focus is on anti–inflammatory, raw, cleansing foods with fiber to help eliminate metabolized estrogen and help prevent PMS symptoms.

- ☐ Eat lots of raw veggies like bell peppers, spinach, jicama, and tomatoes, or lightly steamed, fiber-rich vegetables like asparagus and Brussels sprouts.

- ☐ Incorporate your choice of tropical fruits such as pineapple, papaya, coconut, guava, kiwi, or mango as well as cantaloupe, figs, strawberries, or raspberries.

- ☐ You naturally have more energy during this phase, so go easy on the carbs. Focus on lighter grains like quinoa, amaranth, lentils, or corn.

- ☐ Eat plenty of sesame or sunflower seeds by sprinkling them on salads or smoothies.

- ☐ Anti-inflammatory turmeric (fresh or ground) is also great at this time.

- ☐ If you crave a fresh green juice, go for it. Be sure to choose a raw, organic, cold-pressed, unpasteurized juice with more greens and minimal fruit, or make your own with spinach, dandelion greens, celery, cucumber, apple, turmeric, lemon, and ginger.

Summer Food Chart

VEGETABLES	GRAINS	NUTS AND SEEDS
arugula	amaranth	almonds (almond butter)
bell peppers	corn	pecans
chard	quinoa	pistachios
chives		sesame seeds (tahini)
cucumbers		sunflower seeds (sunflower
dandelion greens		seed butter)
eggplants		
endive	**LEGUMES**	**OTHER**
fennel		
okra	mung beans	chicory
scallions	lentils (any variety)	dandelion tea
spinach	split peas	turmeric
tomatoes		

FRUITS			
apricots	figs	melons	pineapple
cantaloupes	guava	papayas	raspberry
clementines	kiwi	passionfruit	strawberry
coconuts	mangoes		

SUMMER RECIPES

Breakfast

PINEAPPLE TURMERIC SUNSHINE SMOOTHIE

(makes 1 serving)

2 stalks celery, chopped

1 cup frozen pineapple

¾ teaspoon ground or fresh turmeric (or more, to taste)

⅓ cup shredded coconut (unsweetened)

1 scoop vegan protein powder (plain or vanilla)

1-inch chunk peeled ginger

1 tablespoon tahini (can substitute sesame seeds or hemp hearts)

1 cup unsweetened vanilla almond milk + ½ cup filtered water

Handful of ice (optional)

Add all ingredients to a high-speed blender. Blend until smooth.

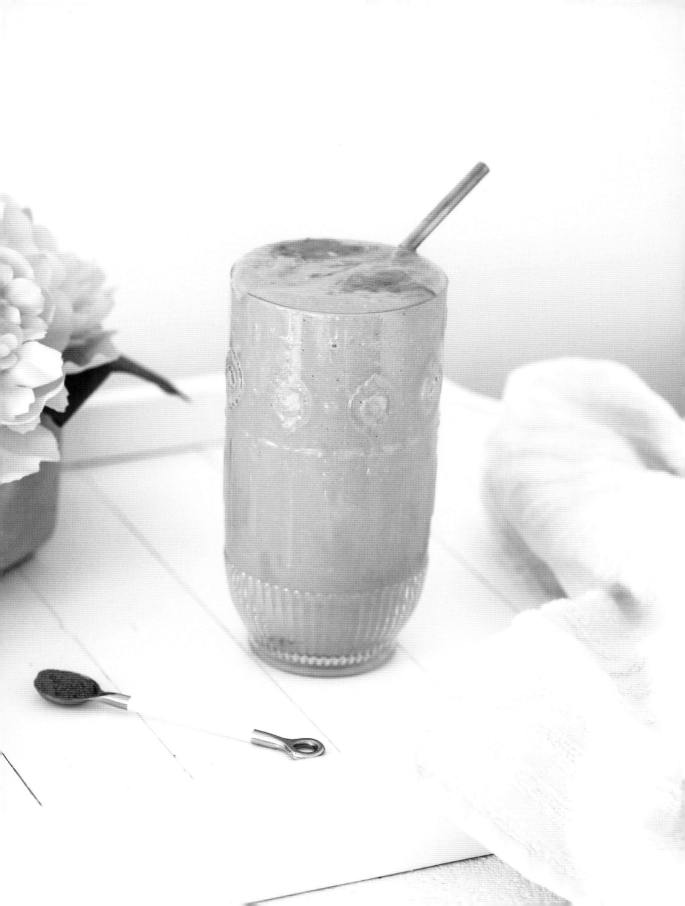

MERMAID DETOX SPIRULINA SMOOTHIE

(makes 1 serving)

2 large handfuls kale (can substitute spinach or dandelion greens)

1 cup frozen mango

½ cup chopped cucumber

1-inch chunk peeled ginger

½ teaspoon spirulina (or more, to taste)

⅓ cup shredded coconut, unsweetened

1 scoop vegan protein powder (plain or vanilla)

1 ½ cups coconut water or filtered water

Handful of ice (optional)

Add all ingredients to a high–speed blender. Blend until smooth.

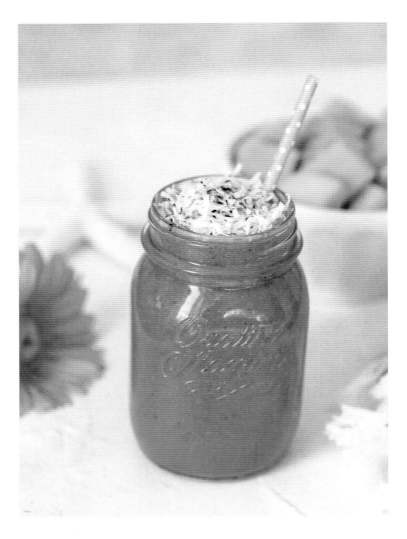

SUMMER LOVIN' OVERNIGHT BREAKFAST JAR

(makes 1 serving)

1 cup light coconut milk
(or unsweetened vanilla
almond milk)

3 tablespoons chia seeds

1 tablespoon tahini (or raw
sunflower seed butter)

½ teaspoon vanilla extract

5-6 stevia drops (or your choice
of natural sweetener)

½ cup chopped strawberries
(or any fruit from the Summer
Food Chart on page 179)

OPTIONAL TOPPINGS:
crushed almonds or
shredded coconut

Combine coconut milk, chia seeds, tahini, vanilla, and stevia in a mason jar. Stir to combine. Let sit one minute then stir again. Add in the strawberries (or summer fruit of choice) and cover with a lid. Refrigerate overnight, or for at least two hours.

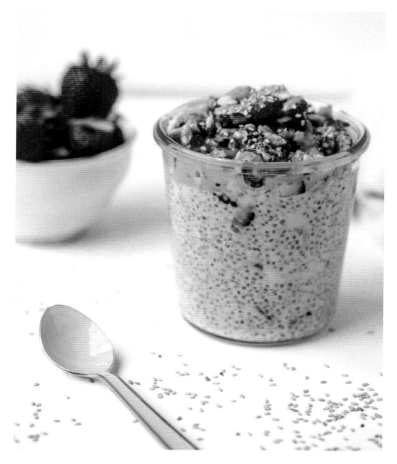

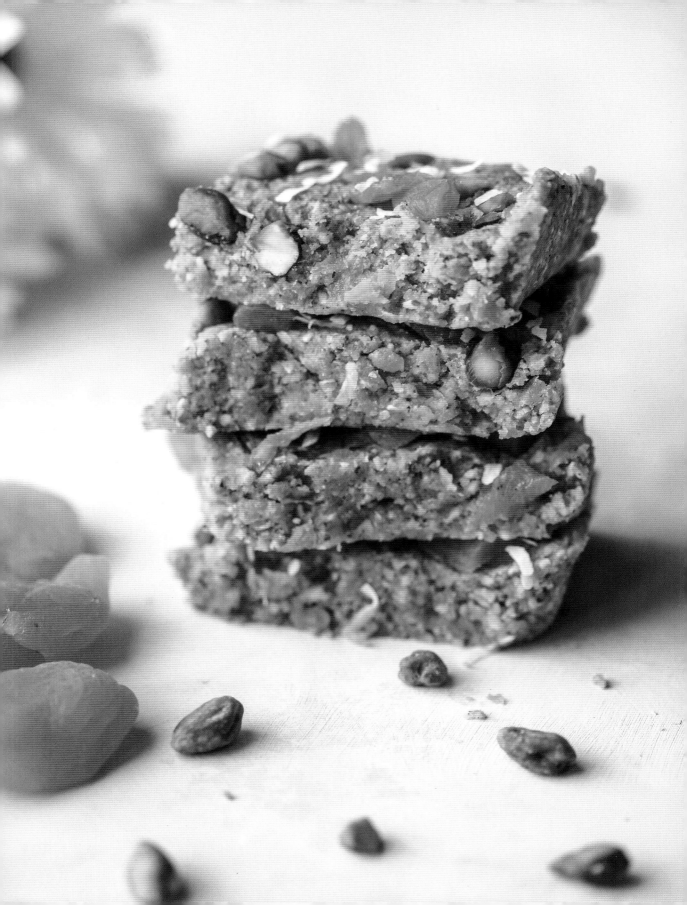

PISTACHIO APRICOT NO-BAKE BREAKFAST BARS

(makes 8 bars—I usually snack on 2 bars throughout the day)

1 cup shredded unsweetened coconut

¾ cup almond flour

⅓ cup shelled pistachios (can substitute raw almonds)

2 tablespoons white sesame seeds

1 scoop vegan vanilla protein powder

Pinch sea salt

1 cup dried apricots

2 tablespoons tahini

1 tablespoon maple syrup

⅓ cup filtered water (or 1–2 tablespoons more if it feels too dry or crumbly)

Combine the shredded coconut, almond flour, pistachios, sesame seeds, protein powder, and sea salt in a food processor. Blend to a fine, crumbly consistency. Next, add the apricots and blend until chopped into small pieces. Add the remaining tahini, maple syrup, and water, and combine until it feels sticky and starts forming into clumps. Press mixture into an 8x8-inch square pan (or a loaf pan if you want thicker bars) and refrigerate for 20 minutes or until firm. Remove from refrigerator and slice into bars; store in the refrigerator.

STRAWBERRY QUINOA MERMAID WRAP

(makes 2-3 servings, 5-6 small wraps total)

1 ½ cups cooked quinoa (or ½ cup dry)

1 bell pepper, chopped (any color)

1 cup chopped fresh strawberries

1 cup chopped cucumber

2 tablespoons fresh parsley (can substitute cilantro)

1 green onion, chopped

3 tablespoons raw sunflower seeds (or sesame seeds)

⅓ cup runny tahini

½ fresh lemon, juiced

½ teaspoon sea salt

5-6 collard leaves (can substitute rainbow chard)

To cook quinoa, combine ½ cup quinoa with 1 cup water in a pot. Bring to a boil, then reduce heat and cover to simmer for 15 minutes or until water is absorbed. In a large bowl, combine cooked quinoa with the remaining ingredients (minus the collard leaves) and stir until well-combined. Assemble about ½ cup of the mixture onto a collard wrap and roll up like a burrito; store leftovers in the refrigerator.

CLEANSING ARUGULA FENNEL SALAD

(makes 2–3 servings)

6 cups arugula

1 small fennel bulb, sliced

2 tablespoons fresh parsley, chopped

2 tablespoons pine nuts (can substitute sesame seeds)

½ cup cooked quinoa

SIMPLE LEMON DRESSING

¼ cup extra virgin olive oil

1 lemon, juiced (about ¼ cup)

1 teaspoon maple syrup

½ teaspoon sea salt

Whisk together the ingredients for the Simple Lemon Dressing in a small bowl, then set aside. In a large bowl, assemble salad starting with the arugula, fennel, parsley, pine nuts, and quinoa. Toss and divide into bowls (or containers to be stored for tomorrow's lunch), then drizzle the dressing.

Note: keep dressing separate for leftovers to prevent the salad from getting soggy.

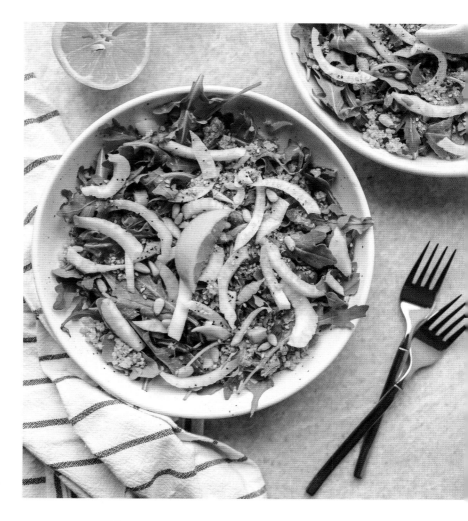

GOLDEN GLOW SUMMERY LENTIL SOUP

(makes 4–5 servings)

2 tablespoons avocado oil (or grapeseed oil)

½ yellow onion, chopped

1 clove garlic, minced

2 teaspoons ground turmeric

2 teaspoons cumin

2 teaspoons ground yellow mustard seed

1 teaspoon ground ginger

1 teaspoon red pepper flakes (optional)

1 teaspoon sea salt

½ teaspoon cinnamon

½ teaspoon black pepper

2 cups broccoli florets

4 cups low-sodium vegetable broth

2 cups light coconut milk

1 ¼ cup yellow mung beans/ split lentils

4 cups spinach

½ lemon, juiced

Heat the oil on medium-high heat in a large soup pot or Dutch oven. Add the onion and sauté 4–5 minutes, until soft and translucent. Stir in the garlic, turmeric, cumin, yellow mustard seed, ginger, red pepper flakes, sea salt, cinnamon, and black pepper. Add in the broccoli and cook for five minutes. Pour in the vegetable broth, coconut milk, and mung beans. Increase heat to high and bring to a low boil, then reduce heat to medium-low to simmer about 15–20 minutes or until mung beans are tender. Turn off heat, then stir in the spinach and lemon. Serve. Store leftovers in the refrigerator (or freeze for up to three months).

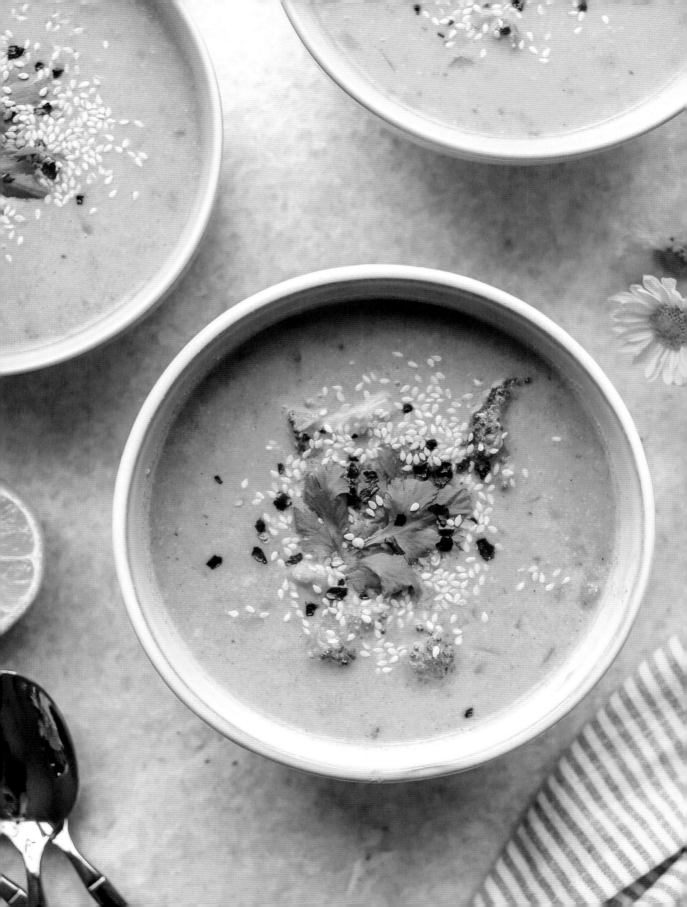

LOVELY LENTILS AND GREENS WITH MANGO SUMMER SALSA

(makes 2 servings)

1 cup cooked lentils any variety,
or ½ cup dry

2 cups arugula (or spinach)

1 ripe avocado,
divided and cubed

MANGO SUMMER SALSA

2 ripe mangoes, diced

1 cup cherry tomatoes, halved

1 fresh lime, juiced

1 can organic sweet corn
(no salt added variety)

¼ cup fresh cilantro

Sea salt and pepper, to taste

To cook lentils, combine ½ cup dry lentils with 1–½ cups filtered water. Bring to a boil, then reduce heat and simmer until tender, about 15–20 minutes. Meanwhile, combine all ingredients for mango salsa in a small bowl and mix. Set aside. When lentils finish cooking, season with salt and pepper; assemble your plate with greens, lentils, mango salsa, and avocado.

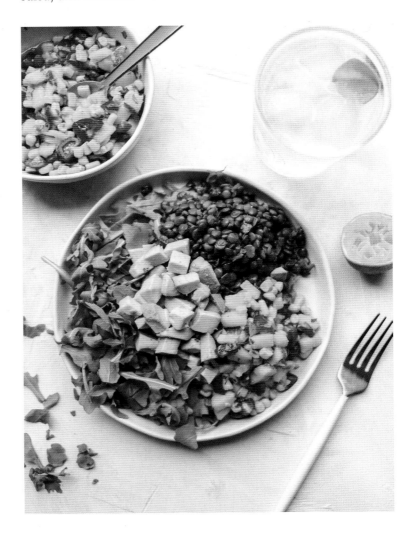

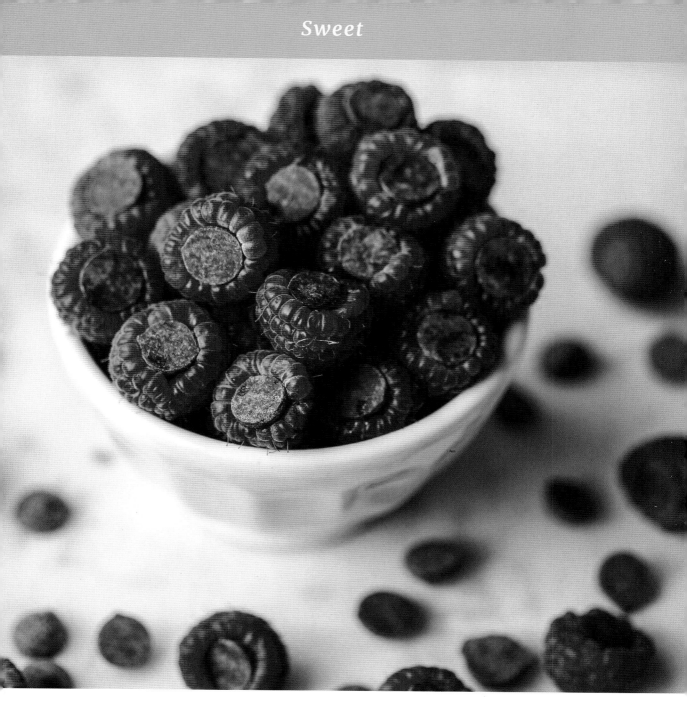

CHOCOLATE-STUFFED RASPBERRIES

1 pint of fresh raspberries

Vegan chocolate chips

Stuff each raspberry with a chocolate chip and freeze or eat a handful as–is; store the remaining in the refrigerator or freezer.

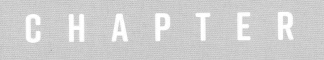

CHAPTER

12

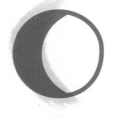

Phase Four:

LUTEAL

Autumn | Waning Moon

LASTS 12-14 DAYS
BBT: 97.7 - 98.3

N AUTUMN, THE LEAVES TRANSFORM INTO BEAU-
TIFUL golden yellow, orange, and red tones before
eventually falling, leaving behind bare branches
that reveal what truly lies underneath. The weather starts
to cool and nature winds down in preparation for the
upcoming winter. Your body acts similarly during this
phase, coming off the energy high from summer (ovulation) as it begins to slow down and prep for hibernation
(menstruation). If your ratio of progesterone to estrogen
is off, or you aren't detoxing estrogen efficiently, you
may start to experience PMS symptoms but remember,
they are not normal or to be expected, contrary to what
you may have been taught. They are merely an indication
of an imbalanced ratio of hormone levels, which you can
gradually restore through the Happy Hormone Method.

The luteal phase is my favorite phase because it's when I get the answers I've been
looking for and gain clarity. Intuition becomes crystal clear. During this time, you
may feel the most detail-oriented, yearning to check things off your to-do list,
finish projects, deep clean the house, and reorganize your entire life and home.
This may also include productive meal prep, catching up on laundry, purging and
donating old clothes, cleaning out the pantry, and running errands that have been
pushed to the side all month. You can thank your rise in progesterone for this. I
find that the luteal phase features my favorite comfort foods.

YOUR HORMONES

This is the post-ovulatory phase when the corpus luteum (what's left of the follicle from which the egg released) transforms into a short-lived endocrine gland and begins producing progesterone, all in one day. The increase in progesterone alerts your body to keep the endometrium (uterine lining) and signals the pituitary to stop releasing FSH and LH, preventing another egg from being released. Progesterone turns the endometrium into a soft bed in case a fertilized egg is implanted for a baby to grow. The ripening of the uterine lining happens every cycle after an egg is released, whether or not the egg fertilizes. Progesterone also stimulates estrogen to rise again, and testosterone to increase slightly before your period arrives. If the egg is not fertilized the corpus luteum is reabsorbed after 12–14 days, and the body prepares for menstruation by stopping progesterone. The drop in progesterone is what triggers bleeding to shed the lining.

Power of Progesterone

Progesterone deserves its shining moment, as it does a lot for the body. While its main job is to maintain and nourish a pregnancy, it also stabilizes your mood (especially in this phase when there could be an excess of estrogen and progesterone will calm you when estrogen levels drop), relieves anxiety, promotes deep sleep, soothes your nervous system, stimulates breast cells to differentiate, and offsets and balances out estrogen, which means lighter periods.

PMS SYMPTOMS AND HACKS

In the two weeks after ovulation and before menstruation, PMS can strike at any time. Hormones are wonderfully beneficial but sometimes, the rise and fall of estrogen and progesterone are too much, and symptoms are inevitable. Especially if estrogen is too high and drops off before or during your period, or when the body is not clearing out excess estrogen and levels are too high in relation to progesterone.

I don't want emotions in the luteal phase to get discredited as hormonal because as women, we are allowed to express our feelings and emotions however we want.

Too often, women are given a demeaning label of being hormonal. While you may feel extra moody, emotional, or weepy during this time, your hormones are not out to get you. What you want to watch out for are any extreme fluctuations or a problem with estrogen detoxification related to diet and lifestyle.

While the following hacks are amazing to combat PMS symptoms, they are meant to use *in addition* to the Happy Hormone Method. The ultimate goal is to eliminate PMS altogether. Until then, try these tips:

BLOATING, PUFFINESS AND DIGESTION ISSUES

☐ **Fennel Tea**: Fennel tea is the one bloating hack I swear by. Whenever I feel puffy or am holding onto water weight, I drink a couple of cups of fennel tea throughout the day, and it works wonders. Fennel supports digestion, reduces bloating, and eases that heavy, too full feeling after a large meal. I drink it 5-6 times per week or as needed throughout the luteal phase. Make sure the tea is of high quality or it won't help with bloat. The brand I trust and prefer for fennel tea is called *Traditional Medicinals*. After steeping, I'll often add 1–2 drops of stevia to sweeten it. You can also combine one fennel tea bag with one ginger tea bag or a licorice tea bag for enhanced digestion support.

☐ **Magnesium Glycinate:** This specific form of magnesium is a *must* for women of all ages, at all times throughout your cycle. Magnesium is an essential mineral responsible for over 300+ chemical reactions in your body. This form is vital for hormone balance, easing bloating, promoting restful sleep, reducing insomnia, and calming anxiety, especially during stressful times as magnesium is the first mineral to be flushed by the body when it's stressed.

☐ **CALM Magnesium Bedtime Tea:** This is a different form of magnesium (the citrate form) but is also a must when digestion is feeling off. This tea is known for calming anxiety. I recommend starting small with a half teaspoon and working your way up to two teaspoons to prevent an upset stomach. Only use it when you are constipated or bloated. Mix the powder into hot water and drink it before bed to wind down. If you take magnesium glycinate every night, reduce it to 200mg when taken alongside the CALM tea.

☐ **Daily High-Quality Probiotic:** Keep your gut flora happy which will, in turn, help eliminate bloating and promote daily bowel movements (see Plant Based Essentials, page 87).

☐ **Leafy Greens:** Increase your intake of steamed, mineral-rich leafy greens (like kale and collards) to help reduce bloating and balance out fluid retention from the high magnesium and calcium concentrations. The increased fiber will promote regular bowel movements.

☐ **Rebounding:** Sometimes our face and bodies feel puffy upon waking, and this can be from a stagnant lymphatic system. Your lymphatic system is an elimination pathway for toxins and fluids that need to expend from the body. When it's sluggish, you may feel the puffiness and extra fluid retention in your face, but it's also throughout your entire body. The only way to drain your lymphatic system is to jump around or move vigorously. Rebounding means jumping on a mini trampoline to help accelerate drainage of lymphatic fluid, by forces of acceleration and deceleration. The up and down motion is beneficial for your lymphatic system since it runs in a vertical direction throughout the body. By gently massaging lymph fluid through the system, it can be pushed out through your lymph nodes and exit the body via urine, bowel movements, or sweat. It is helpful to bounce daily when you feel puffy, and 15-20 minutes should do the trick.

FOR BLEMISHES OR OILY SKIN

You want to make sure your liver is effectively cleansing, breaking down metabolized estrogen, and filtering out toxins. If your liver is not effectively clearing out excess estrogen, it will be eliminated through the next best pathway—your skin—which is the cause of acne and excessive oiliness, especially during the ovulation and luteal phases. To help, I recommend eliminating endocrine disruptors and doing the following:

☐ **Eliminate Sugar:** I owe my clear skin to quitting sugar. I did a sugar detox for four weeks, and my skin has never looked better. I now avoid sugar at all costs (except for fruit and the occasional medjool date). Yes, it was hard at first, and I experienced intense cravings, but I would do it all over again to eliminate blemishes for good. I've noticed a decrease in wrinkles and fine lines, a smoother complexion, and a more even skin tone plus an overall decrease in inflammation (see page 99 for natural sugar alternatives).

☐ **Milk Thistle:** This promotes liver detoxification by drawing toxins out of the body and protecting you from liver damage. Silymarin (derived from the milk thistle plant) has been used in traditional medicine as a natural remedy for liver disease due to its antioxidant and enzyme-promoting activity, increase in bile production, and ability to decrease inflammation. Milk thistle is beneficial after heavy alcohol consumption or long-term prescription drug use. I recommend the *HealthForce Superfoods Liver Rescue Supplement.*

☐ **Exfoliate:** Be sure to gently exfoliate and slough away dead skin, which prevents future blemishes. Using an enzyme cleanser and wet washcloth, remove any impurities. When my skin is feeling extra oily, I turn to the OSEA Cleansing Mudd because it soaks up excess oil and exfoliates without rough ingredients.

CRAVINGS

Intense cravings are all too familiar for me. First, it's chocolate, then salt, and then anything sweet. It feels like a rollercoaster that doesn't stop. Cravings stem from blood sugar imbalance or micronutrient deficiencies and are usually trying to tell you something. Follow these guidelines to address your cravings without going overboard:

☐ If you crave chocolate, you may be low in magnesium, which is why I always keep chocolate on hand because it's full of it. My favorite is ChocZero Dark Chocolate Almond Bark. It's sugar-free and vegan. Lily's also makes vegan stevia-sweetened chocolate bars and chocolate chips, and Addictive Wellness makes suberb high-quality adaptogenic chocolate squares.

☐ If you're craving carbs, it likely stems from a blood sugar imbalance or a vitamin deficiency, which is why I recommend a daily B-complex. It helps curb carb cravings.

☐ If you're craving carbonated drinks, it's possible you are dehydrated. Skip the soda and drink more water.

☐ If you're craving salty foods, you may need to replenish lost mineral stores. Refined salt is stripped of minerals, so it's important you choose the right kind of salt. Start adding sea salt, sea vegetables (like kelp, dulse, or nori) and water-rich vegetables and fruits to your diet (grapes, watermelon, cucumber, celery). They are high on the full spectrum of minerals your cells need. Try my Sticky Water recipe on page 227.

☐ If you're craving something sour, it is likely that your stomach is low in acid. Take a shot of raw, unfiltered apple cider vinegar.

MOOD SWINGS

Keeping your blood sugar balanced with meals that contain high fiber, protein, and fat, and are low in sugar will keep your mood balanced and steady. Roasted root vegetables help as well, as they contain natural sugars that may alleviate the after effects of your estrogen dip which can bring on feelings of anxiousness or irritability. To keep your mood balanced in the luteal phase, I recommend adding more cinnamon to your diet (smoothies, teas, energy balls) as well as making sure to take your vitamin B-complex and magnesium glycinate supplements (see Plant-based Essentials, page 84).

If you experience fatigue or debilitating brain fog, the first thing to do is get a good night's sleep. Manage your stress, limit caffeine and be sure to eat high quality, balanced meals. See Plant-based Essentials for recommended supplements for improved focus and concentration, page 91.

Do You Have Estrogen Excess?

Estrogen excess is the most common hormonal imbalance and is often the main culprit of your pesky PMS symptoms. Long-term estrogen excess (over years or decades), increases your risk of breast cancer and other female cancers, dementia, high blood sugar, and diabetes. Getting your hormone levels tested is preferred to guesswork, but here are some symptoms/conditions that stem from excess estrogen:

- ☐ Fibroids
- ☐ PCOS
- ☐ Endometriosis
- ☐ Ovarian cysts
- ☐ Acne
- ☐ Oily skin and hair
- ☐ Breast tenderness

- ☐ Mood swings
- ☐ Hair loss
- ☐ Feeling puffy/bloated
- ☐ Weight gain before your period
- ☐ Heavy periods
- ☐ Irregular periods
- ☐ Painful cramping

How to Treat Estrogen Excess:

The Happy Hormone Method is the best long-term treatment option for naturally detoxing excess estrogen and balancing your hormonal ecosystem overall, but here are some specific treatment options:

- Detox and nourish your liver with fiber rich foods and liver-supporting nutrients

- Remove endocrine-distrupting chemicals

- Nourish and treat your microbiome health

- Incorporate the Plant-based Essentials (see page 83) and liver-supporting supplements (see page 89)

Do You Have Low Progesterone?

Getting your hormone levels tested using a blood and saliva test is better than guessing whether or not you are low in progesterone, but here are some clues:

- Premenstrual spotting: If you experience brown spotting *before* your first heavy day of bright red colored blood, it may be old blood.

from your previous cycle that has oxidized; this often indicates low progesterone.

- Luteal Phase Defect: If your luteal phase is shorter than 11 days (it should be 12-14 days) this means your corpus luteum did not properly form that cycle, which can cause a progesterone deficiency.

- PMS symptoms in Luteal Phase: If you experience mood swings, irritability, anxiety, bloating, breast tenderness, painful cramps, food cravings, or headaches *before* your period, you may have low progesterone or estrogen excess.

- No rise in BBT mid-luteal phase: If you did not record an increase in temperature in the middle of this phase, it might indicate that you did not ovulate this cycle which means your body will not produce progesterone.

How to Increase Progesterone Naturally

- Balance your blood sugar (see Lifestyle Action Steps, page 96)

- Reduce inflammation (remove sugar, wheat, gluten, dairy, processed vegetable oils, endocrine disruptors)

- Optimize elimination pathways for estrogen detoxification (see page 199)

- Limit or quit alcohol

- Address possibility of HPA Axis Dysregulation by reducing stress (See page 25 for more information on HPA Axis Dysregulation and stress reduction techniques)

- Incorporate the Plant-based Essentials (page 83) and Boost Fertility supplements (page 91)

- Try a natural progesterone cream (made from wild yams) or wild yam extract. It helps bring progesterone levels up but be very careful about your dosage and always talk with your naturopath or doctor before using.

MOOD & ENERGY

Since your natural energy is not as abundant in this phase, you'll feel more drawn to getting your life in order and feeling productive than going out and socializing. Autumn is the transitional season from summer into winter and a time to prepare for hibernation. Aside from checking things off your to-do list, you may feel like taking the time to dive deeper and reorganize what's going on internally with your emotions, intuition, and life. If you sense some internal conflict, don't ignore your inner voice. That is your intuition guiding you to look more closely at something that may need to change, whether it relates to work, relationships, or your social life. You have a heightened sense of awareness and ability to notice things you might have otherwise overlooked earlier in your cycle. These are the superpowers of progesterone. Don't forget to treat yourself to a relaxing bath or curl up with a good book—you deserve it after all of your hard work and productivity in the previous phases.

EXERCISE

This phase lasts for two weeks (10–14 days). During the first week, you might have high energy so continue strenuous workouts from the ovulation phase (hot yoga, strength training, and high-intensity cardio), then start to scale it back with more core-focused workouts like pilates, vinyasa yoga, mat work, and body resistance exercises. You may prefer to workout at home rather than going to the gym. As energy decreases in the second week and you feel more fatigued, choose lower-resistance cardio like the elliptical, bike, walking, or gentle yoga classes. *This is my favorite phase to start streaming the p.volve videos from their website for fine-toning, functional movement training to bring out the natural lines in my legs, stomach, arms, and entire body.*

SEX

You may still feel in the mood during the first week of your luteal phase, but it could take a little longer to get aroused and eventually climax. Work in some extra foreplay and makeout sessions to get you there. Setting up a romantic scene with candles and music can help, too. The same applies during the second week, but you may be more in the mood to snuggle with your partner instead.

LUBRICATION

Following the lubricating fertile mucus in the ovulatory phase, cervical mucus will begin a drying pattern, thanks to progesterone. You may notice it becomes thick, sticky, milky, or even stretchy, but it won't feel slippery anymore. This type of mucus prevents sperm from entering the uterus. It is still considered a wet phase though, so you probably won't need extra lubricant.

SKIN

Estrogen levels drop after ovulation, but then slightly rise with progesterone and fall again before menstruation. Sometimes the fluctuations between estrogen, progesterone, and testosterone in this phase can cause the skin to break out if your body is not detoxing excess hormones properly. Lower levels of estrogen mean less collagen, which can cause the skin to feel less plump and a bit dull. Also, the slight rise in testosterone can lead to thicker sebum (an oily secretion from the sebaceous glands), which can ramp up the oiliness on your skin. A product that works to gently exfoliate, purify, and detox would be beneficial. I like to do face masks 2–3 times per week in the luteal phase, exfoliating to make sure the excess sebum and oil won't clog my pores. This is also the phase when I'm stricter with my morning and night skin care routine, to further prevent breakouts.

DIY AUTUMN FACE MASK

Balancing Banana Mask

1 tablespoon mashed banana

½ tablespoon maple syrup

1 teaspoon coconut milk

½ teaspoon cinnamon

¼ teaspoon nutmeg

Combine all ingredients in a small bowl and mix until well-combined. Apply to clean, dry skin and let sit for 15 minutes. Rinse with warm water and pat dry.

DIY AUTUMN HAIR MASK

Clarifying Baking Soda Hair Scrub

1 ½ tablespoons baking soda (aluminum-free)

1–2 tablespoons shampoo (your regular kind)

3-4 drops tea tree oil (optional)

Mix all ingredients in a small bowl. Wet hair and work the mixture into your scalp and roots, giving yourself a mini scalp massage for 4-5 minutes to slough away product residue and dead skin cells. Rinse thoroughly with warm water and follow with conditioner. *Note: this scrub isn't recommended for color-treated hair.*

FALL ESSENTIAL OIL BLENDS

1–2 drops each, or more as desired

COZY SWEATER: Frankincense, Orange, Nutmeg

FALL MORNINGS: Tangerine and Cinnamon

ANXIETY RELIEF: Lemongrass, Sweet Orange, Ylang Ylang

CRISP FALL AIR: Thyme, Eucalyptus, Lime

PMS-EASE: Lavender, Clary Sage, Ylang Ylang, Cedarwood, Chamomile, Geranium

NUTRITION

- Metabolism speeds up which increases your appetite and cravings.

- Grounding, warming foods like roasted root vegetables and complex carbohydrates can help stabilize the estrogen dip and deter moodiness. They also help curb sugar cravings due to their high amounts of B-vitamins, which help manufacture progesterone.

- Focus on lightly steamed leafy greens or cruciferous vegetables to help the liver flush out excess estrogen.

- Eat foods rich in B-vitamins, calcium, magnesium, and fiber like brown rice, millet, roasted cauliflower, parsnips, squash, or sweet potatoes.

- Choose fiber-rich fruits like apples, pears, peaches, dates, and raisins. Add fresh mint, spirulina, or raw cacao to your smoothies.

- Dandelion tea, fennel tea, and licorice tea help the kidneys flush out excess water to relieve bloat.

- Also, reduce alcohol and caffeine (if you consume it) at this time to decrease inflammation.

Autumn Food Chart

FRUIT	OTHER	NUTS AND SEEDS
apples	cacao (raw/powdered form)	hickory
bananas	cinnamon	peanut (peanut butter)
dates	dandelion tea	pine nuts
jackfruits	fennel tea	sesame seeds
peaches	licorice tea	sunflower seeds
pears	mint	sunflower seed butter
persimmons	peppermint tea	tahini
raisins	spirulina	walnuts

LEGUMES		GRAINS
chickpeas (garbanzo beans)	great northern beans	brown rice
cannellini beans	navy beans	millet

VEGETABLES			
Brussels sprouts	cucumber	mustard greens	shallots
cabbage	daikon	onion	squash (all varieties)
cauliflower	garlic	parsnips	sweet potatoes
celery	ginger	pumpkin	watercress
cilantro	jicama	radishes	yams
collard greens	leeks	rutabagas	

AUTUMN RECIPES

Breakfast

HAPPY HORMONE DETOX SMOOTHIE

(makes 1 serving)

2 cups kale, de-stemmed
(about 2 large leaves)

2 stalks celery, chopped (or ½
cup chopped cucumber)

1 pear, any variety (can
sub an apple)

1-inch chunk fresh
ginger, peeled

Handful of fresh cilantro

½ lemon, juiced

1-½ cups coconut water or
filtered water.

Handful of ice (optional)

Add all ingredients to a high-speed blender. Blend
until smooth.

MOODY MERMAID MINT CHIP SHAKE

(makes 1 serving)

2 handfuls kale leaves

½ frozen banana

1–2 medjool dates, pitted

2 tablespoons cacao nibs

½ teaspoon spirulina

¼ teaspoon peppermint extract

1 scoop vegan chocolate protein powder

1 tablespoon tahini (can substitute raw sunflower seed butter)

1 cup unsweetened vanilla almond milk + ½ cup filtered water

Handful of ice (optional)

Add all ingredients to a high-speed blender. Blend until smooth.

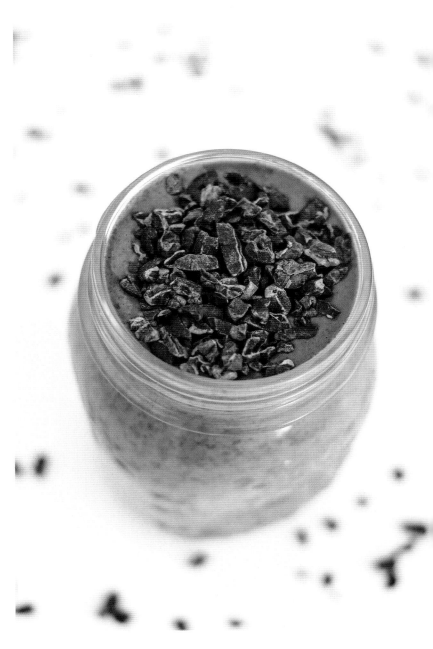

SWEET POTATO TOAST—TWO WAYS

(makes 1 serving)

OPTION ONE

½ sweet potato, sliced thin and lengthwise (¼ inch thick)

1 tablespoon tahini

⅓ banana, sliced

1 tablespoon walnuts

Sprinkle of cinnamon

OPTION TWO

½ sweet potato, sliced thin and lengthwise (¼ inch thick)

1 tablespoon raw sunflower seed butter

3–4 slices of either peach, pear or apple

1 tablespoon raisins

Sprinkle of cinnamon

Place two sweet potato slices in a toaster oven (or regular toaster) and toast on high for five minutes (or longer, depending on your toaster) until soft and cooked through. Add your choice of toppings and serve.

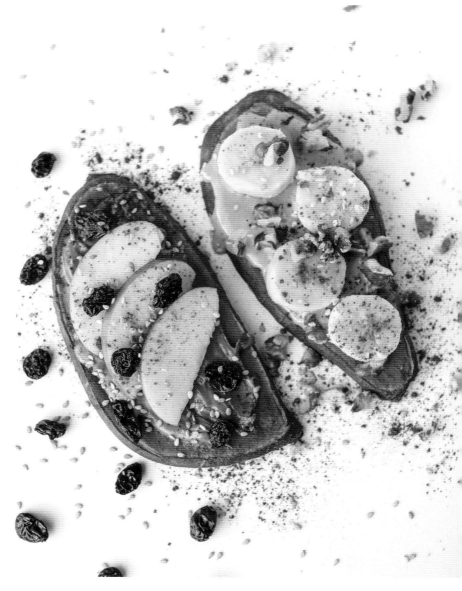

CREAMY PUMPKIN OVERNIGHT OATS

(makes 1–2 servings)

¼ cup gluten-free rolled oats

2 tablespoons chia seeds

½ scoop vegan vanilla plant protein

½ teaspoon cinnamon

½ teaspoon ground ginger

½ cup pumpkin puree (not pumpkin pie filling)

2 tablespoons raisins (can substitute chopped dates for extra sweetness)

1 tablespoon raw sunflower seed butter (can substitute peanut butter)

Stevia, to taste (optional)

1-¼ cup unsweetened vanilla almond milk (or more if too thick)

OPTIONAL TOPPINGS: handful of vegan chocolate chips

Stir oats, chia seeds, protein, cinnamon, and ginger together in a mason jar. Add in the pumpkin, raisins, sunflower seed butter, stevia, and almond milk. Let the mixture sit for one minute and then stir again. Cover with a lid and refrigerate for at least two hours, or overnight.

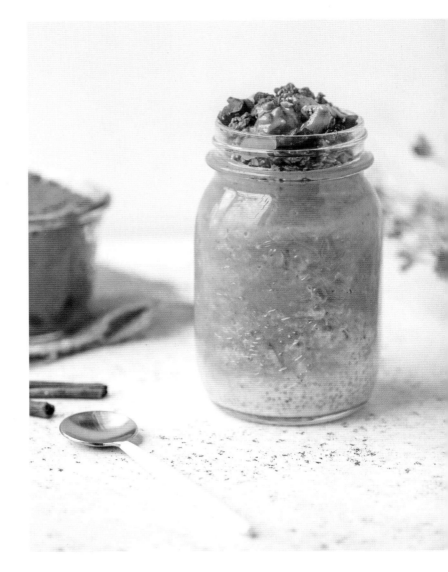

MASHED CHICKPEA SALAD

(makes 2 servings—but I always double the recipe for extra leftovers)

1 cup shredded carrots

2 celery stalks, finely chopped

1 small apple, finely chopped

¼ cup chopped green onion (can substitute red onion)

¼ cup chopped fresh cilantro

1 15-oz can chickpeas, drained and rinsed

2 tablespoons raw sunflower seeds

1 cup chopped kale leaves (can substitute spinach)

2 tablespoons Dijon mustard

2 tablespoons tahini

½ teaspoon minced garlic

½ fresh lemon, juiced

½ teaspoon sea salt

OPTIONAL ADD-INS: raisins, grapes, jicama, radish

Add the carrots, celery, apple, green onion, and cilantro to a large bowl. Set aside.

Add chickpeas to a food processor and pulse a few times until blended, but with chunks remaining for texture (you can also mash in a bowl with a potato masher). Transfer the chickpeas to the bowl with the rest of the ingredients, and mix in the remaining sunflower seeds, kale, Dijon, tahini, garlic, lemon, and sea salt. Taste to test and adjust salt and pepper to your liking. Serve by itself, on toast, with rice crackers, or over greens.

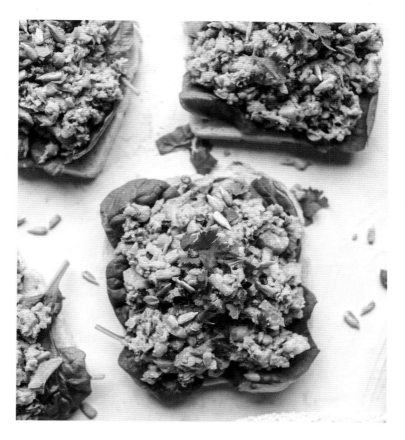

SPICY SWEET POTATO STEW

(makes 4 servings)

2 tablespoons avocado oil (can substitute grapeseed oil)

½ yellow onion, chopped

½ jalapeño, chopped (or more, to desired spiciness)

1 tablespoon freshly grated ginger (can substitute for dried ginger)

1 clove garlic, minced

2 large sweet potatoes, peeled and cubed

1 large zucchini, chopped

3 teaspoons cumin

2 teaspoons coriander

1 teaspoon sea salt

1 teaspoon turmeric

1 teaspoon paprika

½ teaspoon cayenne (optional)

1 28-ounce can diced tomatoes

1 15-ounce can light coconut milk

1 15-ounce can chickpeas (can substitute cannellini beans or Great Northern beans)

2 cups chopped kale leaves (can substitute spinach)

½ fresh lemon, juiced

OPTIONAL TOPPINGS: cilantro, red pepper flakes

Heat oil in a large pot or Dutch oven on medium–high heat. Add the onion and sauté about 4–5 minutes, until soft and translucent. Stir in the jalapeño, ginger, and garlic and cook two minutes. Next, add in the sweet potato, zucchini, cumin, coriander, sea salt, turmeric, paprika, and cayenne. Cook five minutes, then add the canned tomatoes (do not drain the can) and coconut milk. Bring to a low boil, then cover and reduce heat to simmer for 35–40 minutes, or until sweet potatoes are tender. Next, add in the chickpeas and cook for an additional five minutes. Turn off heat and stir in the kale and lemon. Serve alongside brown rice or millet, with toppings of your choice.

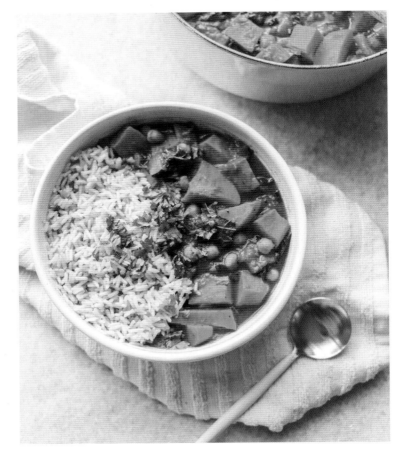

MASHED VEGGIE "POTATOES" WITH CHEESY BRUSSELS SPROUTS AND KALE

(makes 2–3 servings)

1 lb. Brussels sprouts, stems removed and halved

2 tablespoons avocado oil

1 tablespoon nutritional yeast

½ teaspoon red pepper flakes

Pinch of sea salt

1 rutabaga, peeled and cubed (can substitute for 2 parsnips)

1 turnip, peeled and cubed (can substitute for 2 parsnips)

½ head cauliflower florets

Splash of plain unsweetened almond milk (or any plain nut milk)

1 tablespoon refined coconut oil

Sea salt, to taste

2 cups chopped kale leaves

OPTIONAL ADD-INS:
chickpeas

Preheat oven to 400 degrees. Line a baking sheet with parchment paper. Toss Brussels sprouts with oil, nutritional yeast, red pepper flakes, and sea salt. Roast for 20–25 minutes or until crispy.

Meanwhile, bring a large pot filled with water to a boil. After the water boils, add rutabaga, turnip, and cauliflower. Boil for 20 minutes or until veggies are tender. While the vegetables are boiling, steam kale in a pan or small pot fitted with a steamer basket for about five minutes.

When veggies are soft, drain well and add them back into the large pot with almond milk, coconut oil, and sea salt. Mash with a potato masher or a hand immersion blender. Assemble your plate with mashed "potatoes," cheesy Brussels sprouts, and steamed kale.

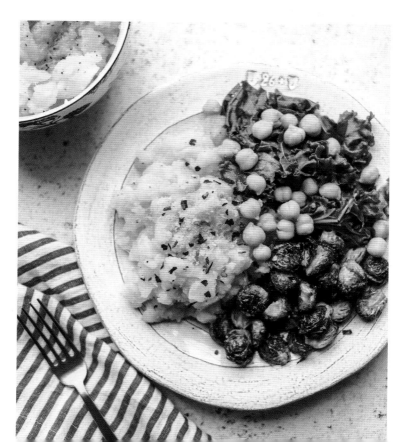

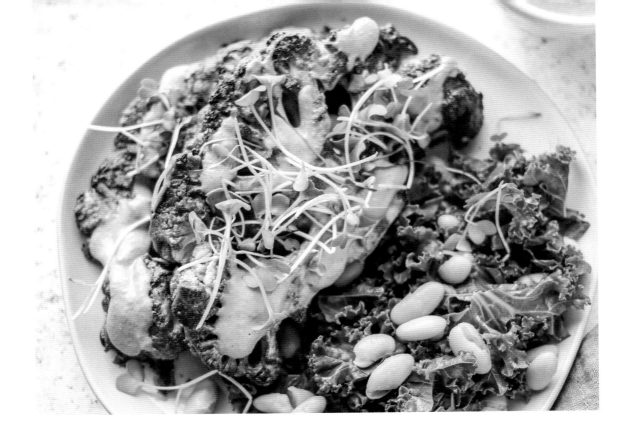

CAULIFLOWER "STEAKS" WITH KALE PESTO

(makes 2 servings)

1 large head cauliflower, cut into 3-4 thick slices

KALE PESTO

1½ cups de-stemmed and chopped kale

½ cup walnuts (can substitute sunflower seeds)

¼ cup nutritional yeast

1 clove garlic

½ fresh lemon, juiced (or more, to taste)

¼ cup extra-virgin olive oil

Sea salt and pepper, to taste

Preheat the oven to 400 degrees. Line a baking sheet with parchment paper.

Remove leaves from the base of cauliflower. Turn cauliflower upside down with the core toward you and cut into three or four one-inch steaks, depending on the size of the cauliflower head. If some of the florets fall off, add them to the baking sheet to be roasted or save them for another recipe. Gently place the cauliflower steaks on the lined baking sheet and slather with kale pesto on each side (about 1–2 tablespoons on each). Save any remaining pesto to use later. Roast for 20 minutes, then gently flip steaks and cook an extra 15–20 minutes, or until golden brown and crispy. Serve alongside greens, cannellini beans or chickpeas.

EDIBLE COOKIE DOUGH

(makes 3 servings)

1 15-ounce can chickpeas, drained and rinsed

½ cup almond flour (can substitute oat or coconut flour)

3 tablespoons sunflower seed butter (can substitute almond butter)

2 tablespoons melted coconut oil

1–2 tablespoons pure maple syrup

2 teaspoons vanilla extract

Pinch of sea salt

2–3 tablespoons unsweetened vanilla almond milk

2–3 tablespoons vegan chocolate chips

Combine all ingredients (except the chocolate chips) in a food processor. Blend until dough forms. Transfer to a bowl and fold in the chocolate chips. Refrigerate leftovers.

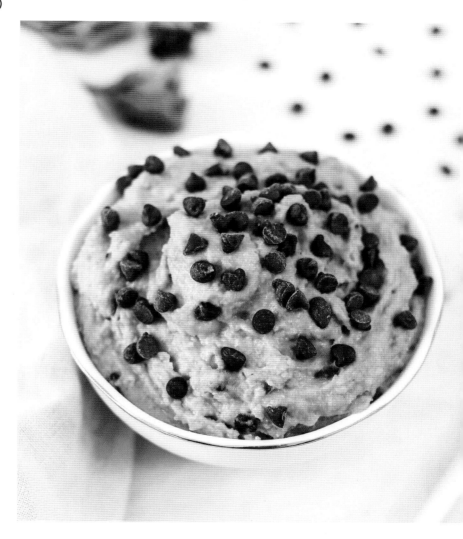

BONUS RECIPES FOR ANY PHASE

"STICKY WATER" AKA HOMEMADE ELECTROLYTE DRINK

(makes 1 serving)

Replenishes lost minerals and electrolytes when you're feeling fatigued or after a sweaty workout.

16 ounces filtered water

Juice of ½ lemon or lime (or more as desired)

1 teaspoon sea salt (I prefer pink Himalayan sea salt)

Combine all ingredients in a mason jar and stir.

GOLDEN TURMERIC LATTE

(makes 1 serving)

1 - ¼ cup unsweetened vanilla almond milk (or any nut milk)

½ teaspoon ground turmeric

½ teaspoon ground ginger

½ teaspoon ground cinnamon

Pinch of black pepper (to help absorb the curcumin in turmeric!)

1 teaspoon maple syrup to taste

In a small pot over the stove, heat and whisk all ingredients together over medium heat until smooth and hot. You can also warm the almond milk in the microwave and then whisk in all the ingredients using a whisk or frother.

SUPERFOOD HOT CHOCOLATE

(makes 1 serving)

1 cup unsweetened vanilla almond milk (or any nut milk of choice)

½ cup filtered water

1 tablespoon pure maple syrup (or raw coconut sugar/cane sugar)

1 teaspoon pure vanilla extract

1 tablespoon raw cacao powder

1 teaspoon raw maca powder

⅛ teaspoon ground cinnamon

⅛ teaspoon ground turmeric

⅛ teaspoon ground ginger

Pinch of cayenne pepper

Pinch of sea salt

Bring the almond milk and water to a slow boil. Then turn off heat and whisk in the maple syrup and vanilla. Combine all remaining ingredients (cacao, maca, cinnamon, turmeric, ginger, cayenne, and sea salt) in your favorite mug. Pour almond milk into the mug and whisk until smooth. Adjust the sweetness level to your liking.

MERMAID LEMONADE

(makes 1 serving)

3 cups filtered water

½ lemon, juiced

1 tablespoon apple cider vinegar (can sub coconut vinegar)

1–2 teaspoons maple syrup, optional (or agave nectar)

¼ teaspoon spirulina powder

Handful of ice cubes (optional)

TIP: *Make sure your water is room-temperature or slightly warm to prevent the spirulina from clumping.*

Pour room-temperature water into a mason jar (or shaker cup) and whisk in all ingredients until well-combined. Add in a handful of ice cubes, if desired. Stir/shake from time to time as the spirulina may settle.

TURMERIC GLOW LEMONADE

(makes 1 serving)

3 cups filtered water

Juice of 1 lemon

½ teaspoon ground turmeric

¼ teaspoon cayenne pepper (optional)

Tiny dash of black pepper (needed to absorb the turmeric)

1 tablespoon pure maple syrup

Handful of ice (optional)

Add all ingredients to a large mason jar and stir until well combined.

GINGER LIME "MOCKTAIL"

(makes 1 serving)

2 tablespoons fresh lime juice

9 ounces sparkling water

6 drops stevia

½ teaspoon grated ginger (use a microplane zester)

Combine ingredients in a jar and stir. Pour over ice in your favorite glass. Garnish with lime.

SEED CYCLING ENERGY BALLS

(makes 10–12 balls)

FOR MENSTRUAL AND FOLLICULAR PHASES

1-¼ cup raw pepitas (pumpkin seeds)

1-¼ cup flaxseeds (raw or ground)

¾ cup vegan plant protein powder (chocolate or vanilla)

½ cup unsweetened shredded coconut

¼ cup raw cacao powder (optional)

Pinch of sea salt

3 tablespoons melted coconut oil

1–2 tablespoons maple syrup (or 10 drops stevia)

1 cup filtered water

In a food processor, combine pepitas, flaxseed, protein powder, coconut, and cacao powder. Blend until finely ground and crumbly. Add in the coconut oil, sweetener, and water, and blend until well combined and the mixture begins to form into one big ball in food processor bowl. Using an ice cream scooper, gently form into balls (the dough is too delicate to roll). Refrigerate for 30 minutes or until firm; store in the refrigerator for snacks or to enjoy alongside your smoothies throughout the week.

FOR OVULATORY AND LUTEAL PHASES

1-¼ cup raw sunflower seeds

1-¼ cup white sesame seeds (I buy these online in bulk)

¾ cup vegan plant protein powder (chocolate or vanilla)

½ cup unsweetened shredded coconut

¼ cup raw cacao powder (optional)

Pinch of sea salt

3 tablespoons melted coconut oil

1–2 tablespoons maple syrup (or 10 drops stevia)

1 cup filtered water

Combine sunflower seeds, sesame seeds, protein powder, coconut, and cacao powder in a food processor. Blend until finely ground and crumbly. Add in the coconut oil, sweetener, and water, and blend until well combined and the mixture starts to form into one big ball. Using an ice cream scooper, gently form into balls (the dough is too delicate to roll). Refrigerate for 30 minutes or until firm; store in the refrigerator for snacks or to enjoy alongside your smoothies throughout the week.

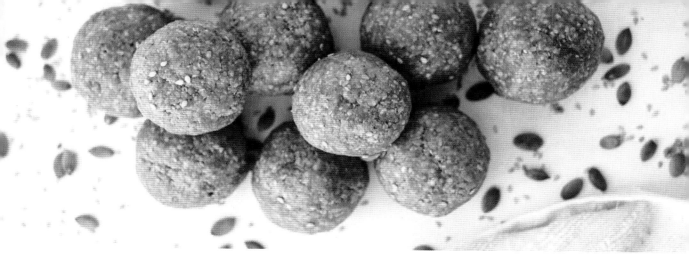

HARMONY CHIA PROTEIN PUDDING

(makes 1 serving)

3 tablespoons chia seeds

½ scoop vegan protein powder

½ teaspoon cinnamon

Vanilla stevia drops (or
2 teaspoons monk fruit
sugar-free sweetener or
coconut sugar)

1 cup coconut or almond milk
(or any nut milk)

1 tablespoon nut
butter of choice

OPTIONAL ADD-INS: cacao
nibs, raisins, berries, granola

Add all ingredients to a jar or bowl and stir until well combined. Wait one minute, then stir again. Refrigerate 1–2 hours or overnight, allowing chia seeds to absorb the liquid and thicken. Feel free to mix in a phase–friendly fruit, too.

HAPPY HORMONE SNACK IDEAS

- ☐ Any fresh veggies from the Food Charts (see pages 133, 156, 179, and 204) to your corresponding phase

- ☐ Any fresh fruit from the Food Charts to your corresponding phase

- ☐ Rice crackers or rice cakes with hummus or avocado

- ☐ Seaweed nori sheets

- ☐ Any nuts or seeds from the Food Charts to your corresponding phase

RESOURCES

ADDITIONAL RECIPES FOR EACH PHASE

I created a phase-friendly recipe section on my blog that categorizes all the recipes I've created into their appropriate phases, so you have plenty more recipe options. I also publish new recipes weekly, so be sure to visit often.

BOOKS

The Period Repair Manual by Lara Briden, ND
WomanCode by Alisa Vitti
Beyond The Pill by Dr. Jolene Brighten
Taking Charge of Your Fertility by Toni Weschler
It Starts With The Egg by Rebecca Fett
The Empowered Woman by Kate Magic
The Hormone Cure by Dr. Sara Gottfried
Sweetening The Pill by Holly Grigg-Spall
No Period, Now What by Dr. Nicola J Rinaldi
The Green Witch: Your Complete Guide to the Natural Magic of Herbs, Flowers, Essential Oils, and More by Arin Murphy-Hiscock
Ask Me About My Uterus by Abby Norman
Women's Bodies, Women's Wisdom by Christiane Northrup, MD
Adrenal Thyroid Revolution by Aviva Romm, MD
Moon Time by Lucy H. Pearce
Wild Feminine by Tami Lynn Kent
Becoming Vegan by Brenda Davis and Vesanto Melina
The Plant-Powered Diet by Sharon Palmer RDN and David L. Katz, MD
Vegan For Her by Virginia Messina and JL Fields
How Not To Die by Michael Greger, MD
Whole by T. Colin Campbell
The Mindful Vegan by Lani Muelrath

WEBSITES

PLANT-BASED LIFESTYLE

chooseveg.com
theveganrd.com
veganhealth.org
happycow.net
vegweb.com
vegansociety.com
findingvegan.com
plantbaseddietitian.com
forksoverknives.com
theglowingfridge.com
mindbodygreen.com

HORMONE HEALTH

drcarriejones.com
fertilityfriday.com
larabriden.com
floliving.com
drbrighten.com
pcosliving.com
healthiernotions.com
nicolejardim.com
amandalaird.com
avivaromm.com
thevaginablog.com
theglowingfridge.com

WOMEN'S HEALTH PODCASTS

Heavy Flow
Fertility Friday
The Period Party
Natural MD Radio
PERIOD podcast
The Holistic Nutritionists
This EndoLife
Hey, Girl
The Fertility Podcast
Hail To The V
The Expectful
Almost 30
Woman Stuff
One Part

HORMONE TESTING

EverlyWell (the Women's Health Test on ever-lywell.com)
DUTCHTest (dutchtest.com)
ZRT Laboratory (zrtlab.com)

APPS

MyFLO tracker
Kindara
Flo
Clue
Glow
Natural Cycles
Ovia
Moody Month
My Cycles
My Moontime – track your cycle with the moon

Ferdy
Happy Cow – for locating plant-based friendly restaurants all over the world. It's especially great when traveling, or to find new veg-friendly spots in your hometown.
Think Dirty – learn the ingredients in your favorite beauty products
Cronometer – track your foods to see where you may be lacking in nutrients

SUSTAINABLE, ECO-FRIENDLY FASHION & CLOTHING BRANDS

Cult of Coquette
In The Soulshine
Joanne Stone
YCL Jewels
Wear PACT
Truth Alone
Vegan Resort Wear
Antidote
LALF
Stormie Dreams
AYNI
HFS Collective
BOTTLETOP

CITATIONS

CHAPTER 1

page 22
Harlow, S.D., Ephross, S.A. (1995). Epidemiology of menstruation and its relevance to women's health. *Epidemiologic Reviews*, 17. Retrieved from https://www.popline.org/node/295425

page 22
Background: Function of the adrenal glands. (n.d.). Retrieved from http://endocrinediseases.org/adrenal/adrenal_what.shtml

page 22
Doll, K.M., Dusetzina, S.B., Robinson, W. (2016). Trends in Inpatient and Outpatient Hysterectomy and Oophorectomy among Commercially Insured Women in the United States: 2000 – 2014. *JAMA Surgery*, *151(9)*, 876-877. doi:10.1001/jamasurg.2016.0804

page 23
Harvard Health Publishing. (n.d.). Understanding the stress response. Retrieved from https://www.health.harvard.edu/staying-healthy/understanding-the-stress-response

page 23
https://www.ncbi.nlm.nih.gov/pmc/articles/PMC4263906/ Hannibal, K., Bishop, D. (2014). Chronic Stress, Cortisol Dysfunction, and Pain: A Psychoneuroendocrine Rationale for Stress Management in Pain Rehabilitation. *Physical Therapy*, 94(12), 1816-1825. doi: 10.2522/ptj.20130597

page 23
Cortisol and Adrenal Function | Dr. James Wilson's AdrenalFatigue.org. (n.d.). Retrieved from https://adrenalfatigue.org/cortisol-adrenal-function/

page 23
Adrenal Function - What Do Your Adrenal Glands Do? (n.d.). Retrieved from https://adrenalfatigue.org/adrenal-function/

page 24
Cadegiani, F.A., Kater, C.E. (2016). Adrenal fatigue does not exist: a systematic review. *BMC Endocrine Disorders*, 16(1), 48. doi: 10.1186/s12902-016-0128-4

page 24
You and your Hormones. (n.d.). Retrieved from http://www.yourhormones.info/glands/adrenal-glands/

page 26
Brain Basics: Understanding Sleep. (n.d.). Retrieved from https://www.ninds.nih.gov/Disorders/Patient-Caregiver-Education/Understanding-Sleep

page 26
Stephens, M. A., & Wand, G. (2012). Stress and the HPA axis: role of glucocorticoids in alcohol dependence. *Alcohol research: current reviews*, 34(4), 468-483. Retrieved from https://www.ncbi.nlm.nih.gov/pmc/articles/PMC3860380/

page 28
Smith, S. M., & Vale, W. W. (2006). The role of the hypothalamic-pituitary-adrenal axis in neuroendocrine responses to stress. *Dialogues in clinical neuroscience*, 8(4), 383-95. Retrieved from https://www.ncbi.nlm.nih.gov/pmc/articles/PMC3181830/

page 28
Andrews, R. (2017, October 03). All About Cortisol. Retrieved from https://www.precisionnutrition.com/all-about-cortisol

page 29
Temperature Regulated by the Thyroid System. (n.d.). Retrieved from https://www.wilsonssyndrome.com/ebook/body-function-dependent-on-body-temperature/temperature-regulated-by-the-thyroid-system/

page 29-30
Thyroid Function Tests. (n.d.). Retrieved from https://www.thyroid.org/thyroid-function-tests/

page 29 and page 31
Negro R. (2008). Selenium and thyroid autoimmunity. *Biologics: targets & therapy*, 2(2), 265-73. Retrieved from https://www.ncbi.nlm.nih.gov/pmc/articles/PMC2721352/

page 31
Ertek, S., Cicero, A.F., Caglar, O., Erdogan, G. (2010) Relationship between serum zinc levels, thyroid hormones and thyroid volume following successful iodine supplementation. *Hormones*, 9(3), 263-268. Retrieved from https://www.ncbi.nlm.nih.gov/pubmed/20688624

CHAPTER 2

page 39
Xenoestrogens: What Are They, How to Avoid Them. (2017, October 26). Retrieved from https://womeninbalance.org/2012/10/26/xenoestrogens-what-are-they-how-to-avoid-them

page 39
Pearson, C. (2013, September 23). Doctors Link Toxic Chemicals And Reproductive Health Problems. Retrieved from https://www.huffpost.com/entry/toxic-chemicals-health_n_3975743

page 39
Toxic Chemicals. (2018, September 04). Retrieved from https://www.nrdc.org/issues/toxic-chemicals

page 39
Vandenburg, L.N., (n.d.). When the dose *doesn't* make the poison: low dose effects & endocrine disrupting chemicals. [Powerpoint Slides]. Retrieved from https://www.efsa.europa.eu/sites/default/files/event/documentset/120614l-p07.pdf

page 42
Neufeld, K., Foster, J. (2009). Effects of gut microbiota on the brain: implications for psychiatry. *Journal of Psychiatry and Neuroscience*, 34(3), 230-231. Retrieved from https://www.ncbi.nlm.nih.gov/pmc/articles/PMC2674977/

page 42

Evans, J.M., Morris, L.S., Marchesi, J.R. (2013). The gut microbiome: The role of a virtual organ in the endocrinology of the host. *Journal of Endocrinology, 218(3)*, R37-R47. doi: 10.1530/JOE-13-0131

page 42

Lobo, V., Patil, A., Phatak, A., & Chandra, N. (2010). Free radicals, antioxidants and functional foods: Impact on human health. *Pharmacognosy reviews, 4(8)*, 118-126. doi: 10.4103%2F0973-7847.70902

pages 42-43

Guinane, C.M., Cotter, P.D. (2013). Role of the gut microbiota in health and chronic gastrointestinal disease: understanding a hidden metabolic organ. *Therapeutic Advances in Gastroenterology, 6(4)*, 295-308. doi: 10.1177/1756283X13482996

page 44

Vandenburg, L.N., (n.d.). When the dose *doesn't* make the poison: low dose effects & endocrine disrupting chemicals. [PowerPoint Slides]. Retrieved from https://www.efsa.europa.eu/sites/default/files/event/documentset/120614l-p07.pdf

page 45

Lymphadenitis 101: What You Should Know About Enlarged Lymph Nodes. (n.d.). Retrieved from https://www.hopkinsmedicine.org/healthlibrary/conditions/infectious_diseases/lymphadenitis_134,80

pages 44-45

MacGill, M. (2018, February 23). Lymphatic system: Definition, anatomy, function, and diseases. Retrieved from https://www.medicalnewstoday.com/articles/303087.php

CHAPTER 3

page 52

Nierenberg, C. (2015, June 30). There's a Sign Women Are Ovulating, But Men Can't Detect It. Retrieved from https://www.livescience.com/51395-sign-women-ovulating-face.html

page 52

Cell Press. (2009, October 8). Unnatural Selection: Birth Control Pills May Alter Choice Of Partners. *ScienceDaily*. Retrieved from www.sciencedaily.com/releases/2009/10/091007124358.htm

page 52

Wenner, M. (2008, December 01). Birth Control Pills Affect Women's Taste in Men. Retrieved from https://www.scientificamerican.com/article/birth-control-pills-affect-womens-taste/

page 52

Berreby, D. (1998, June 09). Studies Explore Love and the Sweaty T-Shirt. Retrieved from https://www.nytimes.com/1998/06/09/science/studies-explore-love-and-the-sweaty-t-shirt.html?pagewanted=all

page 53

Shojania, A.M. (1982). Oral contraceptives: effect of folate and vitamin B12 metabolism. *Canadian Medical Association Journal, 126(3)*, 244-247. Retrieved from https://www.ncbi.nlm.nih.gov/pmc/articles/PMC1862844/

page 53

Palmery, M., Saraceno, A., Vaiarelli, A., Carlomagno, G. (2013) Oral contraceptives and changes in nutritional requirements. *European Review for Medical and Pharmacological Sciences*, 17(13), 1804-13. Retrieved from https://www.ncbi.nlm.nih.gov/pubmed/23852908

page 53

Skovlund, C.W., Mørch, L.S., Kessing, L.V., et al. (2016). Association of Hormonal Contraception With Depression. JAMA Psychiatry, 73(11), 1154-1162. doi:10.1001/jamapsychiatry.2016.2387

page 54

ACOG Committee Opinion No. 651: Menstruation in Girls and Adolescents: Using the Menstrual Cycle as a Vital Sign. (2015). *Obstetrics & Gynecology, 126*, 143-146. Retrieved from https://www.acog.org/Clinical-Guidance-and-Publications/Committee-Opinions/Committee-on-Adolescent-Health-Care/Menstruation-in-Girls-and-Adolescents-Using-the-Menstrual-Cycle-as-a-Vital-Sign

page 54

Garver-Apgar, C. E., Gangestad, S. W., Thornhill, R., Miller, R. D., & Olp, J. J. (2006). Major Histocompatibility Complex Alleles, Sexual Responsivity, and Unfaithfulness in Romantic Couples. *Psychological Science, 17(10)*, 830-835. doi: 10.1111/j.1467-9280.2006.01789.x

CHAPTER 4

page 62

White, A. (2018, December 29). The Greenest Act: A Plant-based Diet. Retrieved from https://www.downtoearth.org/articles/2012-04/2793/greenest-act-plant-based-diet

page 62

Satija, A., Bhupathiraju, S., Spiegelman, D., Chiuve, S., Manson, J., Willet, W., . . . Hu, F. (2017). Healthful and Unhealthful Plant-Based Diets and the Risk of Coronary Heart Disease in U.S. Adults. *Journal of the American College of Cardiology, 70(4)*, 411-422. doi: 10.1016/j.jacc.2017.05.047.

pages 62-63

Reducing Your Footprint. (n.d.). Retrieved from https://www.ewg.org/meateatersguide/a-meat-eaters-guide-to-climate-change-health-what-you-eat-matters/reducing-your-footprint/

page 66

Charles, D. (2014, July 11). Are Organic Vegetables More Nutritious After All? Retrieved from https://www.npr.org/sections/thesalt/2014/07/11/330760923/are-organic-vegetables-more-nutritious-after-all

page 66

Organic FAQs. (n.d.). Retrieved from https://ofrf.org/organic-faqs

page 69

Messina, V. (n.d.). Plant Protein: A Vegan Nutrition Primer. Retrieved from https://www.theveganrd.com/vegan-nutrition-101/vegan-nutrition-primers/plant-protein-a-vegan-nutrition-primer/

page 69

Young, V.R., Pellet, P.L. (1994). Plant proteins in relation to human protein and amino acid nutrition. *The American Journal of Clinical Nutrition, 59(suppl)*, 1203S-12S. http://pilarmartinescudero.es/Ene2018/Plan%20protein%20in%20relation%20to%20human%20protein%20.pdf

page 70

The Plant Plate. (n.d.). Retrieved from https://www.theveganrd.com/vegan-nutrition-101/food-guide-for-vegans/

page 72-73
Vitamins and Minerals. (n.d.). Retrieved from https://www.nal.usda.gov/fnic/vitamins-and-minerals

page 72-73, 84-88
Harvard Health Publishing. (n.d.). Listing of vitamins. Retrieved from https://www.health.harvard.edu/staying-healthy/listing_of_vitamins

page 74 and page 76
Nierenberg, C. (2017, July 21). The Science of Cooking Oils: Which Are Really the Healthiest? Retrieved from https://www.livescience.com/59893-which-cooking-oils-are-healthiest.html

page 77
Hall, A. (2014, April 20). Seed Cycling For Hormonal Balance – Herbal Academy. Retrieved from https://theherbalacademy.com/seed-cycling-for-hormonal-balance/

page 78
Lowcock, E.C., Cotterchio, M., Boucher, B.A. (2013). Consumption of flaxseed, a rich source of lignans, is associated with reduced breast cancer risk. *Cancer Causes & Control, 24(4)*, 813-6. doi: 10.1007/s10552-013-0155-7

CHAPTER 5

pages 84-88
Daily Needs 23. (n.d.). Retrieved from https://veganhealth.org/daily-needs/

pages 84-88
U.S. Food and Drug Administration. (2019). *FDA Vitamins and Minerals Chart.* [PDF File] Retrieved from: https://www.accessdata.fda.gov/scripts/InteractiveNutritionFactsLabel/factsheets/Vitamin_and_Mineral_Chart.pdf

page 86
Aceves, C., Anguiano, B., Delgado, G. (2005). Is iodine a gatekeeper of the integrity of the mammary gland? *Journal of Mammary Gland Biology and Neoplasia, 10(2)*, 189-196. doi:10.1007/s10911-005-5401-5

page 86-88
Greger, M. (2011, September 12.). Optimum Nutrition Recommendations. Retrieved from https://nutritionfacts.org/2011/09/12/dr-gregers-2011-optimum-nutrition-recommendations/

CHAPTER 6

page 99
Mercola, J., Dr. (n.d.). Worse Than Sugar, This Alternative Boosts Your Risk of Obesity and Diabetes. Retrieved from https://articles.mercola.com/sites/articles/archive/2018/05/08/artificial-sweeteners-obesity-diabetes.aspx

page 103
Environmental Working Group. (n.d.). State of American Drinking Water: EWG's Tap Water Database. Retrieved from https://www.ewg.org/tapwater/state-of-american-drinking-water.php

page 105
Xenoestrogens: What Are They, How to Avoid Them. (2017, October 26). Retrieved from https://womeninbalance.org/2012/10/26/xenoestrogens-what-are-they-how-to-avoid-them

page 105
Cleaning Supplies and Your Health (n.d.) Retrieved from http://www.ewg.org/guides/cleaners/content/cleaners_and_health

page 106
Top tips for safer products (n.d.) Retrieved from https://www.ewg.org/skindeep/top-tips-for-safer-products/

page 107
Westervelt, A. (2015, May 05). Research lags on the health risks of women's exposure to chemicals. Retrieved from https://www.theguardian.com/lifeandstyle/2015/may/05/osha-health-women-breast-cancer-chemicals-work-safety

page 108
Black Berkey Purification Elements: Filtration Specifications. (n.d.). Retrieved from https://www.berkeyfilters.com/berkey-answers/performance/filtration-specifications/

CHAPTER 8

page 123
What Is Earthing? (n.d.). Retrieved from https://www.barefoothealing.com.au/v/what-is-earthing/22

page 123
Chevalier, G., Sinatra, S.T., Oschman, J.L., Sokal, K., Sokal, P. (2012). Earthing: Health Implications of Reconnecting the Human Body to the Earth's Surface Electrons. *Journal of Environmental and Public Health, 2012.* 291541. doi: 10.1155/2012/291541

CHAPTER 9

page 128
Price, D.C., Forsyth, E.M., Cohn, S.H., Cronkite, E.P. (1964). The Study of Menstrual and Other Blood Loss, and Consequent Iron Deficiency, by Fe59 Whole-Body Counting. *Canadian Medical Association Journal*, 90, 51-54. Retrieved from https://www.ncbi.nlm.nih.gov/pubmed/14104150

page 130
Weiss, S. (2017, July 21). The Real Reason You Get Horny During Your Period. Retrieved from https://www.bustle.com/p/the-real-reason-you-get-horny-during-your-period-68515

CHAPTER 11

page 172
Pappas, S. (2010, October 17). Booty Call: How to Spot a Fertile Woman. Retrieved from https://www.livescience.com/10828-booty-call-spot-fertile-woman.html

pages 172-173
Reed, B.G., Carr B.R. The Normal Menstrual Cycle and the Control of Ovulation. 2018 Aug 5. In: Feingold KR, Anawalt B, Boyce A, et al., editors. Endotext [Internet]. South Dartmouth (MA): MDText.com, Inc.; 2000-. Retrieved from https://www.ncbi.nlm.nih.gov/books/NBK279054/?report=classic

page 175
Mittelschmerz (Painful Ovulation). (n.d.). Retrieved from http://www.soc.ucsb.edu/sexinfo/article/mittelschmerz-painful-ovulation

ACKNOWLEDGMENTS

I could not have written this book without those who expressed interest in women's wellness. It is you that fueled my imagination and helped me turn an idea into something tangible. Thank you for asking questions, keeping me on my toes, and motivating me to keep learning, sharing, and connecting with the community we've created together. I so appreciate you reading along and keeping up with *The Glowing Fridge*!

To my mom and dad, for the endless encouragement from the very beginning, when no one knew what my little vegan blog could turn into. Thank you for letting me chase my dreams and allowing me to dabble in my passions until I found something that made me happy. Thank you for being there for me no matter what and sharing my blog with everyone you meet!

To my Grandma Shirley, for always steering me to think positively, for helping me to believe that everything happens for a reason, and that everything is going to be okay. Thank you for listening and being a guiding light in my life. You know what I mean, grandma! And to my Grandma June, you are forever missed.

To my love, Terry, for being my biggest supporter of all throughout this process. Thank you for not letting me sulk in my sorrows when I couldn't see an end in sight. Thank you for pushing me to grow stronger and showing me what determination truly looks like. Thank you for not complaining when I hadn't showered for days straight or made you a proper meal for weeks at a time. Most of all, thank you for keeping me laughing and for this amazing life we are lucky enough to share together.

To Elizabeth and Joanie, for always making my recipes, trying everything I blog about and making me feel at home in your sweet family. You don't even know how much your support means to me!

And thank you to my talented photographer Sara, from Sara Hilton Photography, for helping to capture special moments that are sprinkled throughout this book!

To my idols Dr. Lara Briden, Dr. Jolene Brighten, Dr. Carrie Jones, Dr. Chistiane Northrup, and Alisa Vitti for teaching me everything and paving the way for information surrounding female hormone health to be accessible to everyone. Thank you for encouraging women to take their health matters into their own hands, for educating and for offering alternative approaches to women's health matters.

To everyone at Blue Star Press, thank you for believing in me and making this book possible. To Brenna, for being so understanding, compassionate, and helpful throughout the whole process—I will never forget the day I read your email about becoming an author! To Laura Lee for being an amazing editor, and to Alicia, Amy, Amanda, and Peter for bringing everything to life.

INDEX

ABOUT THE AUTHOR

SHANNON LEPARSKI is the founder, photographer, wellness blogger, and recipe developer behind *The Glowing Fridge*, a vibrant blog where she promotes living a plant-based vegan lifestyle. She is a Certified Hormone Specialist through the Institute of Transformational Nutrition. Her passion for wellness, green beauty, and nutrition began in high school and continued through her education at Purdue University. *The Glowing Fridge* has transformed into a plant-fueled resource, allowing Shannon to do what she loves: create vibrant recipes and holistic-based content focused around optimal health and hormone balance. She has inspired thousands to transition toward a plant-forward life! Shannon resides in the northwest suburbs of Chicago with her chihuahua (Taz) and fiancé (Terry).

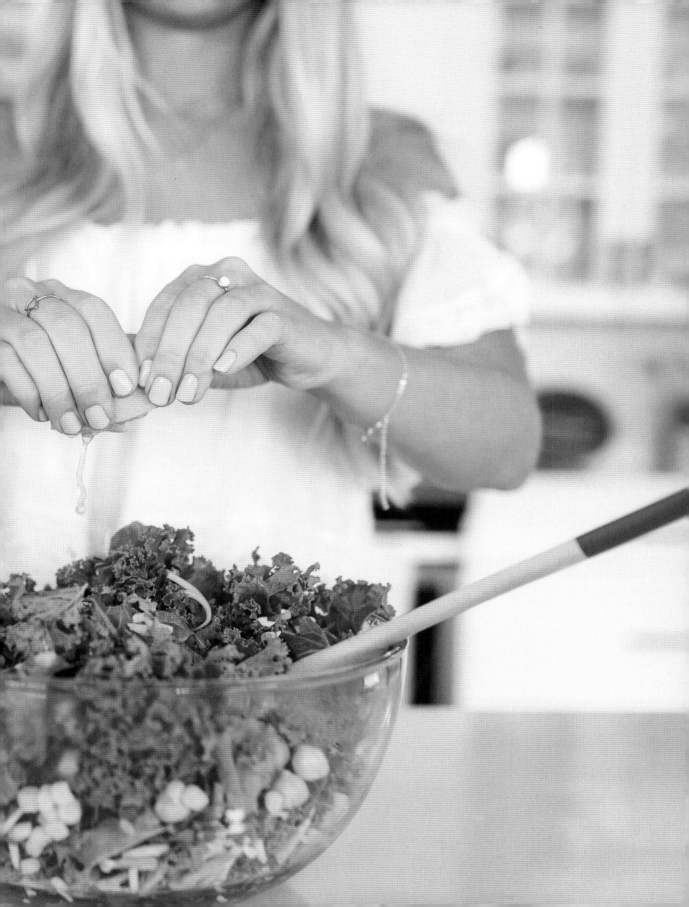